Advanced Technologies and Societal Change

This series covers monographs, both authored and edited, conference proceedings and novel engineering literature related to technology enabled solutions in the area of Humanitarian and Philanthropic empowerment. The series includes sustainable humanitarian research outcomes, engineering innovations, material related to sustainable and lasting impact on health related challenges, technology enabled solutions to fight disasters, improve quality of life and underserved community solutions broadly. Impactful solutions fit to be scaled, research socially fit to be adopted and focused communities with rehabilitation related technological outcomes get a place in this series. The series also publishes proceedings from reputed engineering and technology conferences related to solar, water, electricity, green energy, social technological implications and agricultural solutions apart from humanitarian technology and human centric community based solutions.

Major areas of submission/contribution into this series include, but not limited to: Humanitarian solutions enabled by green technologies, medical technology, photonics technology, artificial intelligence and machine learning approaches, IOT based solutions, smart manufacturing solutions, smart industrial electronics, smart hospitals, robotics enabled engineering solutions, spectroscopy based solutions and sensor technology, smart villages, smart agriculture, any other technology fulfilling Humanitarian cause and low cost solutions to improve quality of life.

Amitava Choudhury · T. P. Singh ·
Arindam Biswas · Mrinal Anand
Editors

Evolution of Digitized Societies Through Advanced Technologies

Springer

Editors
Amitava Choudhury
Department of Computer Science
and Engineering
Pandit Deendayal Energy University
Gandhinagar, Gujarat, India

Arindam Biswas
School of Mines and Metallurgy
Kazi Nazrul University
Asansol, West Bengal, India

T. P. Singh
School of Computer Science
University of Petroleum and Energy Studies
Dehradun, India

Mrinal Anand
Product Security VISA
Austin, TX, USA

ISSN 2191-6853 ISSN 2191-6861 (electronic)
Advanced Technologies and Societal Change
ISBN 978-981-19-2983-0 ISBN 978-981-19-2984-7 (eBook)
https://doi.org/10.1007/978-981-19-2984-7

This Springer imprint is published by the registered company Springer Nature Singapore Pte Ltd.
The registered company address is: 152 Beach Road, #21-01/04 Gateway East, Singapore 189721, Singapore

Preface

The evolution of digital technologies has taken place much quicker than any other innovation in the history of humankind. By penetrating every sphere of life through its powerful reach, it already has transformed the societies and digitized societies which has become a popular phrase to talk about in recent days. Name the area and the impact is felt: may it be education, transportation, connectivity, finances, managing human resources, agriculture, and what not.

In fact, the explosion of information and communication technologies has transformed the way we live, learn, work, and socialize. This heavy intervention of technologies in the modern world has triggered us to think about how we engage and interact with each other and how we make use of these digital tools and communications channels. And consequent upon to this, societies have transformed into digitized societies where datafication, platformisation, and algorithmic governance are common vocabulary words.

This book talks about the evolution of digitization in various spheres of our life and how it became as a part of our social system. In education, for instance, the use of virtual learning platforms opened up the avenues for the students during this extraordinary time of pandemic, and due to technologies only, the teaching-learning remained almost untouched despite the entire world going on lockdown. In the health sector, AI-enabled frontier technologies are helping to save lives, diagnose diseases, and extend life expectancy. Similarly, the presence of digitization in other sectors has been given appropriate space in the book that gives a strong thinking food to the readers. Also, there have been obvious areas where the challenges are due to increased digitization in society like digitally illiterate people; especially senior citizens in the usage of digital technology for improving their life quality and helping them stay in the mainstream of society. These challenges are also addressed at appropriate place in the book. Overall, this is an interesting read for the readers from various backgrounds who are interested in understanding the effect, causes, challenges, and opportunities of digitization in societies.

Organization of the Book

We are delighted to present this book, which was made possible with the support and contributions of academicians from various highly reputable institutions. It is a manifestation of various interesting and important aspects of theoretical and applied research covering complementary facets of innovative algorithms and applications in the fields of digital society, including:

- Introduction to Digital Society: An Overview
- Digitalization of Education-Challenges and Measures for Promotion
- Of Pandemic and Pedagogic Reconstruction: An Epistemological Enquiry into Digital Education in India
- The usage of technology by the senior citizens: opportunities and challenges
- The Phygital Dimension: Redefining Rules of Retail Success through Technological Convergence
- Smart is New Green in Research Evolution
- Role of the fourth industrial revolution towards sustainable development
- An extensive survey focused on smart agricultural based out of IoT
- Globalization of Crime and Digitized Societies: Globalization of Crime and Digitized Societies
- Technology versus Tradition: A human-animal conflict perspective using Game Theory
- Impact of Disruptive Technologies on Society to Combat Pandemic

The very first chapter highlights the concept of Digital Society including features, technologies and components, tools, etc. Digital Society is now not only a concept but also an interdisciplinary research area. In other words, this is a kind of progressive society that has been formed as a result of adaptation as well as integration of advanced technologies into the society and culture. Various subjects and fields become important that are responsible for developing a true Digital Society and these subjects are Information and Communication Technology (ICT), Information Science and Computing, Computer Engineering, etc.

In the second chapter, how education continues during the pandemic is discussed. Since education is a primary aspect to uplift civilization so it must not stop. Hence, all students and teachers although were globally distributed in different places but still education continued locally on time with the help of all these modern communication platforms like email, Google Meet, Zoom, Microsoft Teams, Google Classroom, and many more. Some of the platforms were known to both students and teachers but some were not aware. Thus, it had to be chosen and learnt quickly so that all classes could be conducted within a speculated time and semesters would complete successfully. Here, "Stochastic Hill climbing" optimization technique is implemented to test the success rate of continuous flow of education within time. It is observed that all students could start online classes within a stipulated time along with their corresponding subject teachers. The online classes were conducted on different platforms for taking theory classes and lab classes, providing assignments, and taking examinations. Although different platforms might have been used for conducting different activities, it was solved in an optimal manner.

Recent advances in software and hardware technologies affected the social behavior of human beings a lot. In this progressive world, academics and research are one of the fields that record a massive transformation in terms of delivering the contents to the stakeholders. In addition to technological growth, the impact of COVID'19 while the entire world is in lockdown since the beginning of the year 2020 is highly visible not only in education but in all fields. The COVID'19 exponentially sped up the digital evolution by transporting physical education into digital. Education is one of the research domains where the industrial revolution in the twenty-first century gathered considerable attention. Simultaneously, the infrastructure cost, network connectivity, and digitization are a few of the challenging issues for data transportation from its originator to the end-users. The economical diversity among the population is another criterion to evaluate digitization and digitalization growth and its impact on developing and developed countries. This chapter presents an educational transformation view in a global scenario from digital data to digital platforms.

Then the usage of technology by the senior citizens: opportunities and challenges is discussed along with the real problem definition. This book chapter deals with the opportunities and challenges for the digitally illiterate people; especially senior citizens in the usage of digital technology for improving their life quality and helping them stay in the mainstream of society. The vision of developed India is to make all her citizens literate and it includes digital literacy as well. In general, most of the youth are already digitally literate but somehow, the population in the age group of 50 years and above has only partially achieved it. The reasons may be lack of resources, hesitation in adopting new practices, and fear of cyber frauds due to incomplete knowledge about the processes. Due to these reasons, their life still has not experienced the convenience of the technology. Specifically, in the tough hilly terrains, far-flung areas, villages, and the places having a poor literacy rate, this problem is more severe. Digital literacy is an advantage for senior citizens particularly for those who live alone; live away from their children, grandchildren, and family; and have a desire to stay connected with the family and new world trends. Sometimes, many of them live with mobility constraints but want to live independently in old age. They have to go unnecessarily from place to place, to do tasks, which they can do from their homes only if they know about the appropriate usage of the technology.

The role of the fourth industrial revolution towards sustainable development and how this revolution is widely helpful in progressive digital society are another aim of this book. There are unlimited possibilities when billions of people and devices are connected in real time with unlimited storage, processing power, and access to knowledge. The 4th Industrial Revolution (4IR) is due to technology breakthroughs in wide-ranging fields such as nanotechnology, biotechnology, artificial intelligence, robotics, 3D printing, material science, and high-performance computing, to name a few. 4IR is leading towards a holistic change in industrial sectors and society. New-age computing and automation have long-term implications and replace conventional methods of human interferences in manufacturing, agriculture, and almost all service sectors. These changes will have overlapping effects on workforces. It is, therefore, desirable that the 4IR is sustainable, able to narrow the gap between rich and poor, ensures gender equality, and is beneficial for people in general. 4IR is expected to lead sustainable development goals by promoting regeneration, preservation, and increasing energy efficiency across all industries. New business models may lead to the loss of traditional low-skill jobs and more human-machine interfaces. 4IR should aim at a holistic industrial framework and business model that encompasses technology-driven sustainable growth and empowers people with new skills.

Moreover, how the IoT framework focused on Smart agriculture is another feather of discussion. This study from our research group describes a future IoT using a blockchain paradigm to address these problems. Furthermore, it also offers new ways to encourage creativity. Very energy-efficient cluster assignment integrated approach to IoT agriculture that cuts energy usage and promotes network reliability. Poor-energy adoption clustering level (PEACL) produceS good outcomes. The findings of the simulation demonstrate that the suggested protocol network stability is 24% greater than PEACL as the first node to die in the event of PEACL failure, which occurs at Around 158. IoT-based agriculture begins with the first node's death occurring after 432 cycles. Even still, the energy usage of IoT-based agriculture protocols is 78%. PEACL is lower than that. An extension of the network life to additional rounds, as well as an improvement in network lifetime, is also demonstrated.

Gandhinagar, India — Amitava Choudhury
Dehradun, India — T. P. Singh
Asansol, India — Arindam Biswas
Austin, USA — Mrinal Anand

Contents

Chapter 1
Introduction to Digital Society: An Overview

Amitava Choudhury, Saptarshi Roychowdhury, Binod Kumar Singh, and T. P. Singh

Introduction

The advancement in modern technology along with the human nature of involvement in the procedure of information acquisition and sharing has eased up the way for us to solve the problems in the way of a prosperous society through some fruitful innovations and problem-solving approaches. The researchers, the technologists, the investors, and the device manufacturers all have come up together with joined hands to provide the required technological development and infrastructure to overcome the issues and challenges in information acquisition, structuring, storing, and sharing. Because these are the primitive stages of having a society working with digital information. In the very beginning, it started with the first generation of computers and then evolved into present-day high-end computing. Not only for the computation power, but the area of digital communication has also emerged as a strong and secured field of our modern-day technology. These advancements have not been done in a short span of time, and it has taken quite some lengthy years of research

A. Choudhury (✉)
Department of Computer Science and Engineering, Pandit Deendayal Energy University, Gandhinagar, India
e-mail: a.choudhury2013@gmail.com

S. Roychowdhury · B. K. Singh
Department of Computer Science and Engineering, National Institute of Technology, Jamshedpur, India
e-mail: sap.ratul@gmail.com

B. K. Singh
e-mail: bksingh.cse@nitjsr.ac.in

T. P. Singh
School of Computer Science, University of Petroleum and Energy Studies, Dehradun, India
e-mail: thipendra@gmail.com

A. Choudhury et al. (eds.), *Evolution of Digitized Societies Through Advanced Technologies*, Advanced Technologies and Societal Change,
https://doi.org/10.1007/978-981-19-2984-7_1

and implementation. Now, when we are feeling this wind of change, we are meeting with some stunning technologies like Machine Learning, Internet of Things, and Cloud Computing. These are also the modern computing buzzwords if we consider the latest advancements in computing techniques and which are so much relevant to our digital society concept.

As a cumulative outcome of the tedious and continuous job of the researchers, we can see the transformations from healthcare to e-healthcare, agriculture to smart farming, learning to e-learning, security to smart security systems, etc. We are now relishing the advantages of these new and friendly technology concepts in our day-to-day life, not only in a single sector but distributed among various involvements in our life. Though we believe that we have achieved the society which we call the digitised society, still there are requirements for improvements, and thus, continuous research are going on to make our digital society even better. The motivation of this chapter is to summarise some of the modern research which improve our digitised society by complementing the area of improvements and providing the required solutions for the specific requirements. It is very much demanding that we have to visualise this digitization process in a socio-technical way, and with this continuously evolving technology, our digital society is also bound to be changed rationally. To cope up with this continuously evolving digital society, we also have to be well aware about the facts regarding the required changes that have been made. This chapter will help us to identify and understand the modern state of our digital society from the aspects of the underlying technology.

Overview of Digital Society

In this chapter, as we are discussing about a large-scale area of technology, we have categorised the related research into some different segments e-healthcare, smart farming, e-learning, smart city, smart security systems, etc. In this sector, we try to summarise the latest technological improvements in various sectors of our digital society.

Kart et al. [1] have given an idea of a distributed e-healthcare system for working with the healthcare data in the service-level implementation. This architecture gives a clear vision on how an e-healthcare system provides support to healthcare professionals, as well as patients and patients' monitoring devices. The system is friendlier for the users than existing e-healthcare systems because of its multi-media input and output, which includes text, graphics, and speech.

Hassan et al. [2] proposed a three-tier structure for an efficient fog-based remote pain monitoring system. The fog computing concept is implemented via fog nodes, which are located in the middle tier. The biopotential signals are processed by fog devices, which then send the pain information to web servers via gateway devices.

Ray et al. [3] suggest that industrial standards and aspects of edge computing are critical for the distribution of an improved augmented user experience in conjunction with the Internet of Things. They presented the taxonomical classification and reviewed the industrial factors that can benefit from both the IoT and edge computing scenarios. Secondly, they showed two recently realised use cases that combined the edge-IoT paradigm and urban smart living to solve urban smart living difficulties.

Triantafyllou et al. [4] presented a generic reference architectural model that takes into account a critical non-functional requirement: energy consumption constraints. Furthermore, they explored the technologies that encompass the four tiers of the architecture model: the Sensor Layer, Network Layer, Service Layer, and Application Layer. A discussion of the issues that smart farming monitoring systems confront is also held in this paper.

Dagar et al. [5] examined common agricultural methods used by farmers today and the issues they confront, as well as visited poly homes to learn more about innovative farming technologies. The proposed model is a simple architecture of IoT sensors that gather data and communicate it to a server through a Wi-Fi network, where the server can act based on the data.

Udendhran et al. [6] proposed a method for establishing a safe deep learning system architecture with threat analysis within smart agricultural technologies, which are gaining increasing attention as global food supply needs grow. Smart farming is a combination of data-driven technology and agricultural applications that aids in the production of high-quality food while also increasing crop productivity.

Ali et al. [7] presented an architecture that uses virtual agents to generate semantic suggestions based on user needs and interests, supporting academia in finding acceptable courses in a real-world scenario. When compared to conventional methodologies, the virtualised agent-based recommendation system not only improved user learning capabilities but also made course selection easier, based on users' interests and preferences.

Alfaro et al. [8] offered a software architectural model based on immersive technologies that comprise a description of hardware and software aspects for development and deployment centred on educational activities. The model will allow students to participate in experiences that are very close to reality based on their profiles and characteristics, which were previously identified by a neuro-fuzzy system and treated by a recommendation module, for the generation of experiences and learning objects based on the learning style, resulting in a high degree of personalization in student interaction.

Atawneh et al. [9] proposed that the learner agent, the instructor agent, the device agent, and the social agent are the four components of the proposed model. Because it is responsible for analysing collaborative interactions among various learners, the social agent plays a crucial role in collaborative tasks. It also provides an evaluation indicator for the learners' collaboration and reports on the learners' collaboration with the teacher. A collaborative mobile-learning case study involving two full classes of undergraduate students is used to evaluate the proposed paradigm.

Paul et al. [10] looked into existing threat models and crucial access control issues that deal with multiple permissions on different processing nodes in an IoT context, and it looks for discrepancies. When compared to the existing literature on all security issues, the suggested architecture is comparably efficient in terms of security access control. The primary purpose of this study is to see if blockchain can be used as an alternative to traditional security methods for low-resource IoT applications.

Cha et al. [11] examined how blockchain and Secret Sharing can be used to address privacy concerns in external cloud services and increase data integrity and security by constructing a distributed system. Cloud Service Providers are linked on a blockchain to ensure the integrity of user data and allow easy data access via Transaction. As a distributed system with greater security over existing centralised systems, CSP uses the blockchain to store distributed users' information safely using the Secret Sharing algorithm as a distributed system with improved security over existing centralised systems. Through security analysis, the suggested solution provides greater security and privacy, as well as faster transaction speeds and data storage efficiency than previous research.

Zhang [12] examined the benefits of fog computing and presented a fog-based IoT architecture that efficiently addresses the concerns of huge data processing and network scalability. On this foundation, a layered fog computing network architecture is developed, which uses various intelligence perceptions, information processing, and network transmission means to make the city's operation more coordinated, efficient, and harmonious.

Ray et al. [13] proposed a safe smart home architecture with cloud, secure fog with firewall, and security analysis engine in this study. To defend against illegal data access and Internet risks, the firewall system sits between the Internet and the fog layer. The security analysis engine keeps track of device communication and data transmission and generates notifications for any type of misuse or suspected communication between nodes. This security solution will increase consumer confidence in the use of smart home technology.

Xu et al. [14] presented a Blockchain-Enabled Decentralised Smart Public Safety (BlendSPS) system, which was inspired by blockchain and microservices technology. A microservices-based security mechanism is built using the hybrid blockchain fabric to provide decentralised security architecture, and it supports immutability, auditability, and traceability for secure data sharing and operations across SPS system participants.

Kaul [15] proposed a unique, versatile, technology that is secured on three levels. It is built on locker automation combining RFID technology and software Android App technology, allowing only the bank vault's authorised owner to unlock it. Despite the historical key method, the overall control of the electronic smart door lock system uses RFID tags via NFC, biometric qualities via web portal, and mobile phones via Bluetooth as authentication procedures.

Summary

The literature study shows that various new technologies like cloud computing, blockchain, IoT, digital biometrics, cryptography, etc. have been involved in lots of sections of our digital society. This can be showcased as one of the biggest successes of the human being as it gives the society a better and prosperous future by managing and sharing the gathered information in an efficient manner. The part of the society might be healthcare or farming or education or any other area, and it is now becoming inevitable that to achieve the efficiency we have to invoke these modern technologies into our modern digital society. Researchers are proposing new methods and architectures with which we are getting interacted after the successful implementation of those models. By making a successful implementation of those newly invented technologies, we can surely dream about a successful digital society.

Conclusion

One of the most pressing challenges of our time is the digitalization of society. Digital artefacts and online practises now pervade a significant percentage of our daily organisational, social, and economic activities. Emerging phenomena such as connectivity, platforms, algorithmic power, and big data have a larger scale and scope of revolutionary power than other disruptive innovations in history. This opens up a lot of possibilities, but it also opens up a lot of obstacles. The digitization has lowered the barriers for citizens to participate in problem-solving and innovation to address societal concerns, thanks to technological advancements and a greater openness and culture of involvement and engagement in value creation promoted by the Internet. At the same time, the few infrastructure providers and digital platform owners who enable these activities gain significant power, creating transparency, autonomy, and governance concerns. The Digital Society Initiative is an endeavour to unite researchers in order to contribute to a global digital society that is inclusive, egalitarian, sustainable, and safe, as well as inventive and competitive. In some other debates, digitization also results in a lack of job opportunity for unskilled workers while it raises the job opportunity for the technologists mostly. So, making a large part of the society a better technically abled through some skill development workshops should erase off this negative impact of digitization in socio-economic life.

References

1. Kart, F., Miao, G., Moser, L.E., Melliar-Smith, P.M.: A distributed e-healthcare system based on the service oriented architecture. In: IEEE International Conference on Services Computing (SCC 2007), pp. 652–659 (2007). https://doi.org/10.1109/SCC.2007.2
2. Hassan, S.R., Ahmad, I., Ahmad, S., Alfaify, A., Shafiq, M.: Remote pain monitoring using fog computing for e-healthcare: an efficient architecture. Sensors **20**(22), 6574 (2020). https://doi.org/10.3390/s20226574
3. Ray, P.P., Dash, D., Debashis De: Edge computing for Internet of Things: a survey, e-healthcare case study and future direction. J. Netw. Comput. Appl. **140**, 1–22 (2019). https://doi.org/10.1016/j.jnca.2019.05.005. ISSN 1084-8045

4. Triantafyllou, A., Tsouros, D.C., Sarigiannidis, P., Bibi, S.: An architecture model for smart farming. In: 2019 15th International Conference on Distributed Computing in Sensor Systems (DCOSS), pp. 385–392 (2019). https://doi.org/10.1109/DCOSS.2019.00081
5. Dagar, R., Som, S., Khatri, S.K.: Smart farming—IoT in Agriculture. In: 2018 International Conference on Inventive Research in Computing Applications (ICIRCA), pp. 1052–1056 (2018). https://doi.org/10.1109/ICIRCA.2018.8597264
6. Udendhran, R., Balamurugan, M.: Towards secure deep learning architecture for smart farming-based applications. Complex Intell. Syst. **7**, 659–666 (2021). https://doi.org/10.1007/s40747-020-00225-5
7. Ali, S., Hafeez, Y., Humayun, M., Jamail, N.S.M., Aqib, M., Nawaz, A.: Enabling recommendation system architecture in virtualized environment for e-learning. Egypt. Inform. J. (2021). https://doi.org/10.1016/j.eij.2021.05.003. ISSN 1110-8665
8. Alfaro, L., Rivera, C., Luna-Urquizo, J., Castañeda, E., Zuniga-Cueva, J., Rivera-Chavez, M.:Work in progress: adaptive e-learning software architecture based on immersive technologies. In: 2021 IEEE World Conference on Engineering Education (EDUNINE), pp. 1–4 (2021). https://doi.org/10.1109/EDUNINE51952.2021.9429149
9. Atawneh, S., Al-Akhras, M., AlMomani, I., Liswi, A., Alawairdhi, M., Collaborative mobile-learning architecture based on mobile agents. Electronics **9**(1), 162 (2020). https://doi.org/10.3390/electronics9010162
10. Paul, R., Ghosh, N., Sau, S., Chakrabarti, A., Mohapatra, P.: Blockchain based secure smart city architecture using low resource IoTs. Comput. Netw. **196**, 108234 (2021). https://doi.org/10.1016/j.comnet.2021.108234. ISSN 1389-1286
11. Cha, J., Singh, S.K., Kim, T.W., Park, J.H.: Blockchain-empowered cloud architecture based on secret sharing for smart city. J. Inf. Secur. Appl. **57**, 102686 (2021). https://doi.org/10.1016/j.jisa.2020.102686. ISSN 2214-2126
12. Zhang, C.: Design and application of fog computing and Internet of Things service platform for smart city. Futur. Gener. Comput. Syst. **112**, 630–640 (2020). https://doi.org/10.1016/j.future.2020.06.016. ISSN 0167-739X
13. Ray, A.K., Bagwari, A.: IoT based smart home: security aspects and security architecture. In: 2020 IEEE 9th International Conference on Communication Systems and Network Technologies (CSNT), pp. 218–222 (2020). https://doi.org/10.1109/CSNT48778.2020.9115737
14. Xu, R., Nikouei, S.Y., Nagothu, D., Fitwi, A., Chen, Y.: BlendSPS: a blockchain-enabled decentralized smart public safety system. Smart Cities **3**(3), 928–951 (2020). https://doi.org/10.3390/smartcities3030047
15. Kaul, S.D., Hatzinakos, D.: Intelligent RFID biometric enabled dual security lock in the banking environment. J Bank Financ. Technol. **4**, 159–173 (2020). https://doi.org/10.1007/s42786-020-00022-1

Chapter 2
Continuation of Education During a Pandemic Through Digitalization in an Optimized Manner

Goldina Ghosh and Anwesa Das

Introduction

The education system before the pandemic was in an offline mode where classes were conducted in the classroom using chalk and talk method or PPT presentations. Exams and assignments were totally scheduled and had to be submitted in hard copy, that is, pen and paper method. This mechanism was seen in every school, college and university. Teachers and students had an interaction front to front for classes, examination and problem solving. But a sudden change had to be made when the COVID-19 pandemic took place. Since the modern world is very progressive with all the new technologies, nothing can come to a halt but a slight modification from the normal procedure took place. Hence, this was observed in every aspect of the human race.

The education system has all age groups of people who work in a united manner to perform various activities. A teacher is a person who conveys knowledge to the young generation of the society, who are learners. A very tight but easy bonding must exist between both of these so that the teacher can teach the students and the students can learn the concepts easily. For this reason, a set of rules and regulations are always prepared and maintained by each institute to run the curriculum successfully. The mode of teaching is always a two-way communication. Thus, these entire phenomena are very easy and possible when everybody is physically present in an institute within a particular classroom and interactions take place front to front.

G. Ghosh
Department of Computer Science & Applications, Institute of Engineering & Management, Salt lake, Kolkata, India
e-mail: goldina.ghosh@iemcal.com

A. Das (✉)
Department of Computer Science & Applications, Institute of Engineering & Management, Salt lake, Kolkata, India
e-mail: anwesa.das@iemcal.com

A. Choudhury et al. (eds.), *Evolution of Digitized Societies Through Advanced Technologies*, Advanced Technologies and Societal Change,
https://doi.org/10.1007/978-981-19-2984-7_2

Now suddenly conducting these phenomena in an online mode while keeping the standard of education as it is was a real challenge. Some of the common observed challenges were

(1) Lack of flexibility in the mode of conducting a class;
(2) Technical issues present in online mode;
(3) Lack of interaction with some students missing in online mode;
(4) Presence of immediate feedback to solve problems;
(5) Monitoring each student in virtual mode was difficult especially for practical classes;
(6) Shortage of efficient learning due to complex communication processes.

Although all these difficulties were present, still it was observed that the continuation of education was possible through digitalization in an optimized manner. Here in this research work, it was observed that the transformation of offline to online classes suddenly was possible by using the entire existing modern platform as a medium for continuing with the regular classes, assignments and exams. The research work focuses on this concept by testing the success rate of a continuous flow of education within time through "Stochastic Hill Climbing" optimization techniques.

The remaining part of the work has been arranged in the following manner. Section 2.2 contains the related work section, and the details about the methodology are in Sect. 2.3. Section 2.4 contains the preparation of the dataset which is followed by the result and discussion in Sect. 2.5. Conclusion is in Sect. 2.6.

Related Works

It is highlighted that transformation digitally in the education system changes the modern world rapidly; this is very encouraging for a teacher as well as a student to get involved in the new technology and become a qualified user of the new digital platforms [1]. Online learning is replacing the traditional classroom with virtual teaching such that students can study whatever they want to be a part of their classes, and the class is attended from anywhere at any time with a communication virtually [2]. The education system connects with scientific and technical development and is transformed into it. The introduction of online learning introduces distance learning using digital technology which helps the communication part between student and teacher at any distance. It is important that all types of students of all classes and teachers can understand how the technology works which is used for their classes for easy access. The learning management system (LMS) is also implemented. But sometimes it may hamper the regular classes and routine [3, 4]. Sometimes, the e-examination system was not perfectly implemented. But day-to-day communication, everyday practice and after that examination is highly necessary for students to gain knowledge from teachers. So, the necessity of the digital process is to be consistent but not reduce the utility of the normal teaching-learning process. It forces the digital system to be more easily accessible to all users. It is true that the changes in the system have a huge effect on the normal life as well as education. But education should not be stopped. With the help of new technology, we can go forward in education also [5, 6]. Advanced digital technology like various platforms should be an easy option for users. In the field of digital education, some inclusion and exclusion have been done and developed with online platforms. Many qualified and competitive research works specify the need to search the new option for the online education system with the help of the framework of progressive development and restructuring of older options for teaching like redefining the role of teacher, and the role of students via an online platform. In this regard, the interest is attracted to the topic of changes in the educational system that occurs under the influence of digitalization [7]. As a teacher or as a student, a meaningful way that builds skill is very much needed. To gain digital literacy, an integral part of the system should be in a more natural way. Some core component is required in this regard to maintain professional communication virtually and that should be consistent always. More than one source and justification of all assignments related to study are required. It is also required that students and teachers both are technically knowledgeable [8–10]. With this component, the issue of attendance in online classes should not be affected. The attendance system on a regular basis should be monitored and the status of it should be in a good position for every class. Some good quality approach has been applied when the attendance is monitored via online platforms [11, 12]. In recent days, various types of research works are done on the online method of a teaching-learning environment which is going under the pressure of COVID-19. This disease hampers the normal mode of teaching and learning. So, a smooth way of conducting the process in online mode is highly necessary [13, 14]. Various types of platforms like Zoom, Google Meet, Google Classroom, MS Teams, Blackboard and many more are under research for smooth progress. Sometimes, an integration of a few methods is designed and makes all the components easy for quality education. Teachers as well as students display their satisfaction and dissatisfaction when designing their required course using those platforms [15–17]. All the disciplines should be considered when reviewing all the components like conducting classes, exams and giving some assignments. Some advantages come when reviewing—the timetable of teaching and learning is flexible, physically location change is not needed, interaction between teacher and students has no time bound and less stress of time management [18]. Especially for medical students, video conferencing classes are really well-accepted. Teachers and students both appreciate some components of online platforms [19]. But it has some disadvantages too. The concentration, self-discipline and isolation are really very disappointing. Some students are not able to keep their concentration and interest on the subjects which they are practicing [20]. So, the platforms which are used should be more user-friendly and acceptable to those users. For successful teaching in online mode, all users should be satisfied with all the components [21]. Research and survey are the requirements to get the optimal solutions in this field. In the field of digitization, many complex algorithms have been used with some explained models which are used to survey the effect of education systems to expand the access to knowledge through virtualization in education [22–24]. The Hill Climbing algorithm is one of the popular algorithms for optimization in modern technology. Hill climbing, a mathematical method, considers a heuristic value and optimizes all possible results. The algorithm belongs to the concept of searching technique locally. Stochastic hill climbing is a variant of the hill climbing algorithm. As no one can avoid practicing through digital learning, it should be in an optimal mode. Through some simulations, the way of learning has been changed a lot [25–27].

The motivation of this work is to analyze some popular platforms which are used in online mode for the future improvement of the online process. The effective evaluation of all constraints is highly required. Initially, the survey was done on various platforms with some teachers and students. The data is collected from the responses to fetch a good result regarding the entire platform's utility.

Dataset

In order to carry out the experimental work and observe the results, a dataset preparation was essential. An initial survey was made among the teachers and students to select the platform for conducting classes. Some of the selective platforms that were chosen based on some properties like how many participants can join, what the mode of joining is, if there is a mode of using a whiteboard or a PPT can be presented, platforms that can share materials with the attended participants, authentication of the participants, platforms that provide the facilities for giving and collecting assignments and conducting exams and many more. Among all the platforms presented, some of the familiar suggested platforms recommended by the school/college authorities, teachers and even students were taken under consideration for testing and finally coming to a decision of choosing a platform for conducting classes. Some of the recommended online platforms were "Zoom", "GoToMeeting", "MS Teams", "Google Meet", "Google Classroom", "TCS iON Digital Learning", "Cisco Webex" and "Blackboard Collaborate".

Here for the research purpose, the dataset consists of 300 students (200 males and 100 females) and 20 teachers (11 males and 9 females) of a particular institute. The recommended platforms were put to a survey. The survey was done by both the teachers and students to understand its applications and how fast it can be learnt and adopted. The optimal platform for both students and teachers was chosen based on two primary characteristics. Students and teachers spent the day studying the platform and then voting "For" or "Against" the platform. This was done so that the platform with the best number of votes in less number of days could be selected. The results are presented in Table 2.1. Table 2.1 contains the name of the platforms used with the corresponding number of days the survey was complete with the voting results.

Table 2.1 Survey record

Platform used	Number of days for survey	Voting number (out of 320)	
		For	Against
Zoom	2	246	74
GoToMeeting	4	150	170
MS Teams	5	193	127
Google Meet	3	202	118
Google Classroom	3	197	123
TCS iON Digital Learning	5	168	152
Cisco Webex	4	187	133
Blackboard Collaborate	5	143	177

Table 2.2 Voting ration report

Platform used	No. of days for survey	Ratio of voting (For:Against)
Zoom	2	123:37
GoToMeeting	4	15:17
MS Teams	5	193:127
Google Meet	3	101:59
Google Classroom	3	197:123
TCS iON Digital Learning	5	21:19
Cisco Webex	4	187:133
Blackboard Collaborate	5	143:177

Another record is shown in Table 2.2 which contains the voting ratio of "For" and "Against" values by teachers and students with respect to the number of days for the survey for the same applications.

Methodology

To perform the analysis, the work has been visualized from the concept of solving problems by searching techniques. Since the intention was to find out an efficient online platform for conducting online classes, a perfect searching methodology was implemented to find the success rate of a continuous flow of education within time. For this reason, the Stochastic Hill Climbing searching algorithm was implemented. This algorithm chooses randomly those values from the uphill moves and provides better solutions.

There are certain procedures that need to be maintained before implementing the algorithm. Firstly, the problem and its target solution need to be described. So, the proposed problem and its desired solution are described below.

Well-Defined Problems with Their Solutions

The problems and their corresponding solutions can be defined with the help of the five components using a searching mechanism. They are "Initial State", "Actions", "Transaction Model", "Goal Test" and "Path Cost". In order to start defining the problem, the states need to be discussed then the five components need to be derived. Thus, the states and the five different components as per the research work are as follows:

States: Digital platforms that could be used for conducting online classes.

Initial State: Any randomly chosen digital platform for finding the suitability of its performance.

Actions: Study the use and utility of the digital platforms within a stipulated time and give a vote for it.

Transaction Model: Selecting the corresponding platform for conducting classes, giving assignments, study materials and taking examinations.

Goal Test: Could the chosen platform fulfill the purpose of the online class requirements?

Path Cost: Within a less time period, the platform was easily understandable and could fulfill all the desired outcomes, and had the majority votes in its support.

Stochastic Hill Climbing Algorithm

Stochastic Hill Climbing algorithm is a type of Hill Climbing algorithm. It is also an optimization algorithm where the neighbor is chosen randomly, and a decision is made whether to choose it as a current state or choose another neighbor randomly. The algorithm is as follows.

```
Stochastic Hill Climbing Algorithm
Input: Identify Initial State, Current State
Output: Declare Goal state

Start
  Evaluate the Initial State
  If Initial State is Goal State then
        stop and return success
  else declare Initial State as Current State

   For i=1 to n
     If solution is success || Current State does not change then
          Select a state randomly from the neighbor of Current State better than Current State
      If chosen state is Goal State then
          return success
      else make it as Current State and repeat
   End for
Stop
```

Analysis as Per the Stochastic Hill Climbing Algorithm

It is to be detected that less time with maximum votes is taken for choosing the particular digital platform for conducting the classes successfully. It is denoted by Eq. 2.1

$$vote \propto \frac{1}{time} \tag{2.1}$$

It is to be detected that the voting rate is high within a short period of time. This denotes that the particular platform was easily understandable by both teachers and students. Thus, that particular platform could be chosen for conducting online classes.

According to the algorithm, it is required to check the corresponding condition tallies with Eq. 2.1. Here, Eq. 2.1 will give the goal state value.

To choose the next nearest neighbor in the else condition, Table 2.1 is sorted in ascending order. Again, the values are compared with Eq. 2.1 values.

The steps are repeated until the correct set of the satisfying result for choosing the digital platform is selected.

Results and Discussion

The target of the research work was to prove that although the educational system got a drastic transformation from offline to online mode, the system was not hampered. All teachers and students adapted to the new normal mode of digital education. Days were less, and which platform to choose to carry on with the educational system

Table 2.3 Final survey report

Platforms used	Number of days for survey	Positive response
Zoom	2	246
Google Meet	3	202
Google Classroom	3	197
Cisco Webex	4	187
GoToMeeting	4	150
MS Teams	5	193
TCS iON Digital Learning	5	168
Blackboard	5	143

smoothly was a big challenge. Hence, things had to be planned in an optimal manner. This has been observed and proved.

To start the analysis, certain initial observations were made. From the values in Table 2.1, it is observed which platforms took less days for the survey. The results have been displayed in Table 2.3. According to the number of days for survey and positive response, it is observed that "Zoom" had the first priority for conducting classes and Google Meet had occupied the second position, and this platform was used for providing study materials, giving and receiving assignments and also for conducting semester exams.

The graphical representation is given in Fig. 2.1. In Fig. 2.1, it is observed that eight different platforms were selected for choosing the best one with less number of days. The lists of minimum days taken for the survey are as follows:

"Zoom" takes the least amount of time for analysis, just 2 days, and "Google Meet and Google Classroom" take 3 days.

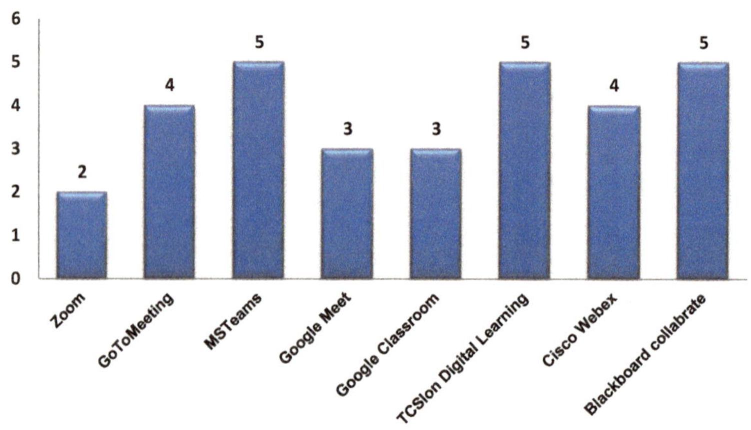

Fig. 2.1 Survey report as per the number of days

Now, not only the number of days but also the rate of votes obtained by each platform was important. "For" and "Against" are the two attributes observed in Table 2.1. From there, the graphical analysis is observed in Fig. 2.2. From this graphical analysis, it is distinctly observed how many platforms got the maximum number of votes as "For "and how many "Against".

A closer and distinct analysis is made in terms of the "For" and "Against" voting values. The rate of difference is sometimes too high and sometimes too less for each of the platforms. This has been observed in Fig. 2.3. In this figure, both the "For" and "Against" values are plotted to denote the marginal differences in the voting values.

In Fig. 2.4, the analysis is done between two important parameters—Number of days of response and Positive response. Different platforms have different times (in

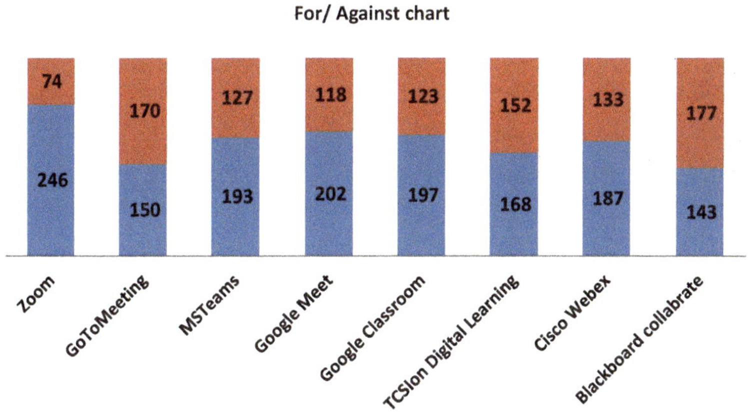

Fig. 2.2 For/Against chart

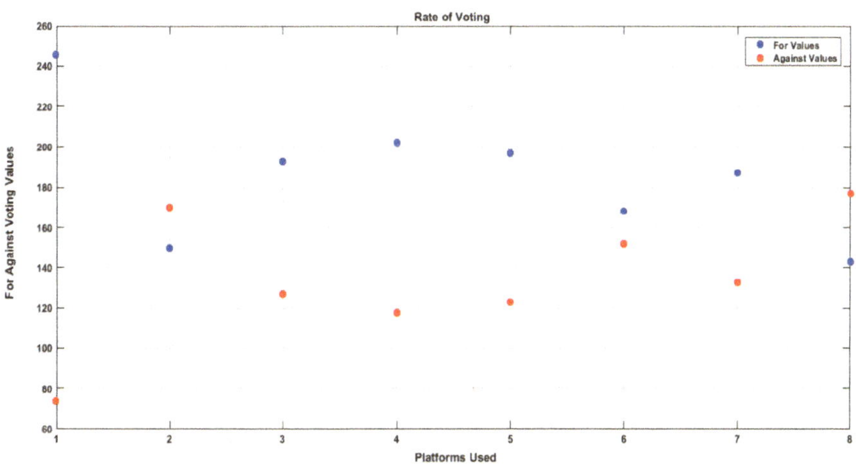

Fig. 2.3 Rate of voting difference between "For" and "Against" values

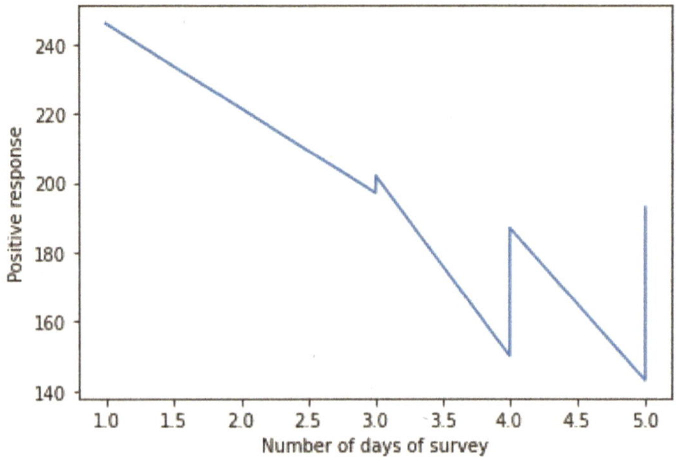

Fig. 2.4 Relation between "Positive response" and "Number of days of survey"

days) of the survey as well as positive responses. From the graph, we can see that if the number of days is increasing, the positive response is decreasing or vice versa. We can tell that these two parameters are inversely proportional to each other as per our database. From this analysis, Zoom has the max positive response with the minimum number of days of survey and Blackboard has the minimum positive rate with a maximum number of days of the survey among those platforms according to our database.

Conclusion

Currently, our focus is on the schools and colleges in cities and towns but for villages, a very close investigation needs to be made. Since the Internet facility is not so high as compared to the cities and towns conducting classes in online mode, might have been difficult. According to the analysis done in this experimental work a distinct observation was made that although the educational system changed from offline to online mode drastically, the flow of education continued with the help of digitalization. A very quick survey had to be done to choose the best platform for conducting classes, giving study materials and conducting exams. To fully fill all these activities within time was a challenge. The whole work was done in a very optimal manner. This has been justified with the Stochastic Hill Climbing algorithm. The concept of inverse proportionality was implemented to select the best platform. Maximum votes in less number of days were the target to accomplish the experimental work. The results obtained focused on two different attributes, i.e., less number of days for the survey and getting maximum votes in support of using that platform. After doing the analysis, it was seen that the "Zoom" platform got the maximum number of votes in fewer days. It received 246 votes in 2 days. This platform was used for conducting classes online. Another platform that was chosen for conducting classes was "Google Meet" as it had received 202 votes in 3 days. Next for giving study materials and conducting exams, "Google Classroom" was chosen as it had obtained 197 votes in 3 days. Thus, a clear view was given in the form of tables and graphs. Although this survey was only made from city and town schools and institutes, for further analysis the survey can be extended to village schools and institutes to detect what conditions they went through. This will help in getting a complete view of the continuation of education during a pandemic through digitalization in an optimized manner.

References

1. Larisa, K., Anna, L., Nataliya, G., Yana, A., Organization of higher education in context of digitalization: online learning experience at pandemic, development trends. In: E3S Web Conf., vol. 273, pp. 12052 (2021). https://doi.org/10.1051/e3sconf/202127312052
2. Artur, V.K., Pecherista, E.V., Kirillov, A.T., Aleksandra, V.C.: Current problems of higher education development in the Russian Federation considering the digitalization processes. In: Conference (SPBPU IDE '19), St. Petersburg, vol. 38, pp. 1–7 (2019). https://doi.org/10.1145/3372177.3373341
3. Alexander, J.M.: Learning to Save the Future: Rethinking Education and Work in an Era of Digital Capitalism. (2018). https://doi.org/10.4324/9781315450209
4. Vanya, D.: Digitization of Education in the Field of Security. International Conference on High Technology for Sustainable Development (HiTech), pp. 1–3 (2018). https://doi.org/10.1109/HiTech.2018.8566554
5. Daniela, P., Angela, R., Daciana, L., Mariana, N., Claudiu, C.: Using mixed methods to understand teaching and learning in COVID 19 times sustainability, MDPI. Open Access J. **12**(20), 1–20 (2020). https://doi.org/10.3390/su12208726
6. Deng, X., Zhou, G., Xiao, B., Zhao, Z., He, Y., Chen, C.: Effectiveness evaluation of digital virtual simulation application in teaching of gross anatomy. Ann. Anat. Anat. Anz. **218**, 276–282 (2018). https://doi.org/10.1016/j.aanat.2018.02.014
7. Allsop, S., Hollifield, M., Huppler, L., Baumgardt, D., Ryan, D., Van Eker, M., Spear, M., Fuller, C.: Using videoconferencing to deliver anatomy teaching to medical students on clinical placements. Transl. Res. Anat. **19**, 100059 (2020). https://doi.org/10.1016/j.tria.2019.100059
8. Rasheed, R.A., Kamsin, A., Abdullah, N.A.: Challenges in the online component of blended learning: a systematic review. Comput. Educ. **144**, 103701 (2020). https://doi.org/10.1016/j.compedu.2019.103701
9. Cervi, L., Tornero, J.M.P., Tejedor, S.: The challenge of teaching mobile journalism through MOOCs: a case study. Sustainability **12**(13), 5307 (2020). https://doi.org/10.3390/su12135307
10. Hodges, C., Moore, S., Lockee, B., Trust, T., Bond, A.: The difference between emergency remote teaching and online learning. EDUCAUSE Rev. (2020)
11. König, J., Jäger-Biela, D.J., Glutsch, N.: Adapting to online teaching during COVID-19 school closure: teacher education and teacher competence effects among early career teachers in Germany. Eur. J. Teach. Educ. **2020**(43), 608–622 (2020). https://doi.org/10.1080/02619768.2020.1809650
12. Saul, D., Steinmetz, G., Lehmann, W., Schilling, A.F.: Determinants for success in climbing: a systematic review. J. Exerc. Sci. Fit. (2019). https://doi.org/10.1016/j.jesf.2019.04.002
13. Velev, D., Zlateva, P.: Virtual reality challenges in education and training. Int. J. Learn. Teach. **3**(1), 33–37 (2017). https://doi.org/10.18178/ijlt.3.1.33-37

14. Olszewski, B., Crompton, H.: Educational technology conditions to support the development of digital age skills. Comput. Educ. **150** (2020)
15. Crompton, H., Bernacki, M., Greene, J.A.: Psychological foundations of emerging technologies for teaching and learning in higher education. Curr. Opin. Psychol. **36**, 101–105 (2020). https://doi.org/10.1016/j.copsyc.2020.04.011
16. Burbules, N., Fan, G., Repp, P.: Five trends of education and technology in a sustainable future. Geogr. Sustain. **1**(2), 93–97 (2020). https://doi.org/10.1016/j.geosus.2020.05.001
17. Tilhou, R., Taylor, V., Crompton, H.: 3D virtual reality in K-12 education: asystematic review. In: Yu, S., Ally, M., Tsinakos, A. (eds.) Emerging Technologies and Pedagogies in the Curriculum. Springer, New York, NY (2020)
18. Hodges, C., Moore, S., Lockee. B. et al.: The difference between emergency remote teaching and online learning. EDUCAUSE Rev. (2020)
19. Varea, V., González-Calvo, G., García-Monge, A.: Exploring the changes of physical education in the age of COVID-19. Phys. Educ. Sport. Pedagog. 1–11 (2020). https://doi.org/10.1080/17408989.2020.1861233
20. Skaalvik, E.M., Skaalvik, S.: Teacher stress and teacher self-efficacy: Relations and consequences. In: McIntyre, T., McIntyre, S., Francis, D. (eds.) Educator Stress. Aligning Perspectives on Health, Safety and Well-Being, pp. 101–125. Springer, Cham (2017)
21. Burns, R.: A COVID-19 panacea in digital technologies? Challenges for democracy and higher education. Dialogues Hum. Geogr. **10**(2), 246–249 (2020). https://doi.org/10.1177/2043820620930832
22. Varea, V., González-Calvo, G.: Touchless classes and absent bodies: teaching physical education in times of COVID-19. Sport. Educ. Soc. 1–15 (2020). https://doi.org/10.1080/13573322.2020.1791814
23. Finley, S.M., Conflicts in communication and academic needs for virtual education gifted students. Honors Undergraduate Theses, vol. 879 (2021)
24. Fermín-González, M.: Research on virtual education, inclusion, and diversity: a systematic review of scientific publications (2007–2017). Int. Rev. Res. Open Distrib. Learn. **20**(5), 146–167 (2019). https://doi.org/10.19173/irrodl.v20i5.4349
25. Al-Azawei, A., Parslow, P., Lundqvist, K.: The effect of universal design for learning (UDL) application on e-learning acceptance: a structural equation model. Int. Rev. Res. Open Distrib. Learn. **18**(6), 54–87 (2017). https://doi.org/10.19173/irrodl.v18i6.2880
26. Gunjan, N.: Professional development through virtual education and training. Int. Rev. Res. Open Distrib. Learn. **2**(5), 394–397 (2015)
27. Zogheib, B., Rabaa, A., Zogheib, S., Elsaheli, A.: University student perceptions of technology use in mathematics learning. J. Inf. Technol. Educ.: Res. **14**, 417–438 (2015)

Chapter 3
Digital Transformation in Education

Customary to Digital Education

Amit Singh

Introduction

The customary education system that started from gurukul, madarsa, and the church is now converted into highly modernized classrooms equipped with all digital gadgets. This transformation is distributed consistently over three decades if the last one year of the COVID-19 pandemic is ignored. The upthrust of COVID-19 on digitization and digitalization in education is measurable and people feel that the world has advanced a decade after the COVID-19 stage. The change in teaching–learning pedagogy and the motivation of digital transformation encourages students to better understand with the feel of education which was missing for the last few decades [1].

At the same time when education is progressive in the direction of digitization and digitalization, the challenges like gadget security, infrastructural cost, and most importantly immature behavior of kids, and youngsters are becoming a huge concern to the guardians. In addition to this, the paradigm shift of mindset from the traditional education system to digitize modern education is also not easy for both the instructors and students. However, nothing is permanent, the change is the law of nature and the demand of the current generation leads to the development of digital resources. Here are two terms, i.e., digitization and digitalization [2] discussed above and that need to be clarified more before moving forward:

Digitalization [3–5]: It is a process of using digital platforms and equipment. Transporting physical work of execution into digital technologies. A few examples of such gadgets are computers, laptops, pads, etc.

A. Singh (✉)
School of Computer Science, University of Petroleum and Energy Studies, Dehradun, Uttarakhand 248011, India
e-mail: amit10jul1980@gmail.com

A. Choudhury et al. (eds.), *Evolution of Digitized Societies Through Advanced Technologies*, Advanced Technologies and Societal Change,
https://doi.org/10.1007/978-981-19-2984-7_3

Digitization [6–8]: As far as digitization is concerned, it is a process of converting physical documents into binary format commonly known as the encoding process.

These two terms are different but usually both can be seen simultaneously. The reason for this is the support of both is required to transform a physical system into a digital system. Digitalization is a process of transforming the physical things into digital, whereas digitization is converting physical things into binary and that can be observed over a digital platform of equipment. Hence, without digitization, we are not able to realize or experience digitalization.

The requirement of a pretty beautiful campus and maintaining infrastructures is not an easy task. Can we replace it with a virtual classroom where presentation needs to improve virtually that looks pretty good but does not exist physically? If we can assume this way of teaching and learning process, it leads to digitization and digitalization of physical processes and documents. The purpose of this modernization is to emphasize on connections and interactions among kids and adults irrespective of the level of the studentship and thus motivate them for the teaching–learning.

Before going ahead, let us first discuss the challenging problems faced and prospects [9] of such a system in terms of the stakeholders (i.e., industry, guardian, and students):

Advantages Over the Customary Education System

Although the impact of a paradigm shift in education from customary to the digital world is beyond comparison. The customary and digital education has their own pros and cons along with challenges. A few of the advantages are listed below [10]:

(i) More than only learning about concepts and things can be accomplished through the use of digital devices and digitized content. It interestingly provides the feel and part of the content to the students.
(ii) The most important is the infrastructure and its maintenance cost can be reduced drastically.
(iii) The commute time can be reduced and students can access the educational content anywhere round the clock. The digitized contents can be accessed in rural as well as urban areas effectively and the *right to education* can be achieved for everyone.
(iv) As the earth's ecosystem is considerably and unintentionally destroyed by human beings for the cause of the well-being. However, somehow digitization and digitalization may contribute a lot to the reconstruction of the ecosystem that can ensure sustainability due to the fewer construction requirements.
(v) The knowledge can be transferred to new upcoming generations. Hence, preserving the old physical documents is essential for the future ahead. It is one of the dimensions that can be addressed by digitizing the existing physical documents.

The above are the few measure highlights that can be revoked the welfare of mankind and sustainable development.

Challenges in Transforming the Education System

The issues in digitization and digitalization in the education sector are based on the skill transformation and to change the mindset. Further, it is based on the age group of aspirants and can be summarized as follows:

(i) Primary education is the schooling of kids that is mostly based on the fundamental knowledge of values, manner skills, social practices, basic sciences, environment, and initial level of politics to build the thinking capability among the students. This category of students is the growing and learning stage of their age. While equipping these students with digital gadgets, such as computers, laptops, and mobile phones for education and learning, the risk of distracting them with the content of crime, adulteries, gaming, and flaws of social media at the same time. Another challenging issue is the availability of resources with the economically challenged guardians who cannot afford gadgets and minimum required high-speed internet.

(ii) Secondary schooling students are in the 10th and 12th grades, and they are more prone to being distracted by adulterous knowledge before reaching adulthood. It is extremely harmful and necessitates increased parental and school attention.

(iii) Higher education reflects the graduation and post-graduation standards and requires high-end digital gadgets and infrastructures. In addition, designing such content and delivering it to students as per their easy consumable capacity is different for different segments of students.

(iv) Only the interested and sincere students are utilizing the internet-based online education while most kids and teenagers are misusing the resources and getting involved with unfair content. Moreover, the guardians must be aware of the basic knowledge of online teaching–learning so that they can keep on track of the ward. This basic understanding of parents is another challenging issue with the online or blended mode of education.

(v) Another challenging area is the digitization of available content [11]. A huge amount of study content available worldwide needs to be exported in binary format and regular modification is required to make it more appealing and interesting to the participants.

(vi) A huge amount of storage capacity is demanded by such large databases. As the storage requirement of high definition audio, video, text, and images, etc., is increasing day by day, is another dimension to think about.

The measure points mentioned above are the few challenges in the transformation of education. However, a long list along with the change of mindset of students and experts needs to be synchronized with the new system of the digital era.

Conventional to Modern Education: Digitalization and Digitization

As mentioned above in the chapter, digitalization is the process of presenting physical things over digital gadgets. The growth and investment of the digital market has expanded exponentially in the last few years. The digital equipment connects people with the content and gets the feeling as part of the content of interest. In this section, some of the digital Learning Management Systems (LMS) required for education are explored and tried to understand the fundamental requirement in the concerned sector.

Educomp: Educational Communications

An Indian-based private limited company *"Educomp"* was established in 1994 and created a path for the twenty-first century's online teaching–learning process [12, 13]. Further, the company expanded its educational digital products and solutions across international borders like the United State of America, Singapore, etc. The fundamental incorporation of the company was to convert the customary education system to digital-equipped virtual classrooms and somehow the company achieved this goal (*Smart_ClassTM* launched in 2003). In addition, the company has launched *"Online Tutoring"* for a few specific subjects to transport the physical tutoring to a technology-enabled virtual tutoring system. Educomp has provided technology-enabled solutions to the kids of kindergarten to 12th standard.

The purpose of the Educomp company is to set up the business under the *BOOT model (build, own, operate, transfer)* and manage the private and Indian government schools and laboratories. An education online portal *"PlanetVidya.com"* was launched by the company to spread the business as well as digital education transformation.

Although the company Educomp is currently suffering from an economic fall, it has provided upthrust to the digital transformation of the Indian education system. It has mapped the traditional curriculum into 2D–3D digital content to arouse the interest level of the learners.

Blackboard: A Learning Management System

Blackboard is a learning management system that can be used by teachers and learners for assignments, quizzes, tests, and online synchronous and asynchronous classes [14]. A study is carried out about the effectiveness of blackboard in Saudi Arabia for English as a Foreign Language (EFL) instructors over university-level students [15]. The results of the study were average and the instructors and students realized few pros and cons in the LMS. However, people feel that the proper understanding and few due medications can be an efficient solution of digital education. In the survey, it has been found that 75% of participants faced issues as new in the system and never used the digital LMS priory. A few of the points mentioned below are the highlights of blackboard LMS [16]:

(i) Creating new courses and their management allows teachers to initialize and update the course as per the self and student's need.
(ii) Accessing the calendar and setting due dates of different events are other promising features that can automate the education system, and thus enrich the digital transformation in the education sector.
(iii) Blackboard connects users to the emailing and notification system that can track the activities happening.
(iv) Similarity check is one of the best features that can ensure academic integrity among the users and thus, promotes fair evaluation.
(v) Connecting and accessing the internet makes it more user-friendly for the teachers as well as students to go through unlimited availability of content.

In addition to the above, grading of students, tracking of content accessing, online submission of activities provide a complete digital platform to monitor, teach, evaluate and grade students. However, A study cum survey was conducted and used sentinel analysis to understand the effectiveness of blackboard over different categories of users [17]. It found that there is some issue at students' end, whereas it is appreciated at the instructor level.

MOODLE: A Course Management System

MOODLE (Modular Object-Oriented Dynamic Learning Environment) is a free package designed from the customary pedagogy to support digital education [18]. It is open-source software licensed under GNU general public license norms. It gives flexibility to anyone who freely uses, modifies, and distributes others but cannot change the basic GNU license. The most important feature of moodle is that it can plugin other software as per need. Some of the features are given below [19]:

(i) MOODLE supports learning by observing peers' activities.
(ii) It can be customized by the administrator as per the need of the instructors and students. The full log can be accessed by the instructor and also visible to the students.
(iii) Instructors can set timelines for different activities and also monitor the students to meet expectations.
(iv) It supports cooperative learning, such as wiki, blogs, forums, etc., so that the teacher and students can interact socially and collaborate their learning.

MOODLE as a course management system is a powerful and user-friendly tool for virtual teaching–learning but it has some issues while EFL writing and is highlighted in [20]. Another study on EFL reading effectiveness of students through the MOODLE platform is conducted and found better than the customary instruction-based education system [21].

The impact of LMS on the teaching–learning process is analyzed in [22]. The authors have discussed different patterns of the students' involvement, different parameters are selected to study the different segments of students, and the relationship between the students' pattern and final marks obtained. An LMS-based e-learning system is designed in [23] for vocational education and a research is carried out over 15 undergraduate students of the age group 22–25. The author claims a higher level of satisfaction than the customary education system.

Along with the old LMS system, new machine learning techniques are being applied to enhance the usability and performance of LMS [24]. The data analytics are proposed using Artificial Intelligence (AI) to improve the recommendation of courses and certifications to the students as per their interest and history. The application of Artificial Intelligence-based techniques is further critically reviewed and analyzed in [25, 26] that opens another dimension of research in this field to understand the student mindset.

MOOCs [26]: Higher Education Support—Edx, Coursera, Alison, and NPTEL

As Internet and Communication Technology (ICT) increases day by day, the students of higher education are required to have access to study material over different platforms. The online open-access and open-source MOOCs provide a huge amount of study material [27]. The most widely used open-access platforms Edx [28], Coursera [29–31], and Alison [32] are utilizing the internet services and attracting students by world-class instructors. Similarly, the Indian government initiative for e-learning, an open-courseware NPTEL [33] is started for engineering students throughout the globe.

The features of such online platforms are mentioned below:

(i) These MOOCs provide the best world-class instructors from different universities and colleges around the globe.
(ii) In addition to the study material and asynchronous lectures, they access students for their level of knowledge.
(iii) Such MOOCs provide certification for the course that is valid in so many universities and colleges to compensate for the students' course credits.
(iv) Thousands of students throughout the globe can access the online MOOC courses anytime, anywhere over different digital devices. Hence, mobile education is promoted by MOOCs.

All MOOCs have their pros and cons in terms of their business model and compatibility with the learners and teachers [34, 35]. However, it plays a significant role in digital transformation when it comes to the education sector and need to be nurtured in a better shape.

Recent Software Advancement in Education

Although online education was started long back, the recent COVID-19 pandemic accelerated at a great pace. When all the institutions and universities throughout the globe are not operating offline, the only way to continue education is online mode. Hence, lot of software platforms, such as zoom, google meet, Microsoft teams, etc., are initiated and carried out to support students from kindergarten to higher education [36]. These tools are compatible with operating systems like Windows, Linux, Android, iOS, macOS, etc. Some of the software tools are discussed in this section for online meetings and conducting virtual classes.

ZOOM is one of the cloud-based proprietary software developed by Zoom Video Communications [37]. It offers free plans as well as subscription-based plans and allows up to 1000 participants at a time for 30 h of duration. Banking, industry, healthcare, distance education, remote work meetings, and discussions can be accomplished through zoom effectively. However, the weak authentication issue of zoom compromises security and privacy. To address the authentication issue, a Photo Response Non-Uniformity (PRNU)-based camera authentication is proposed in [38] for online teaching and meeting, and results are validated for small-sized classes.

Similarly, Google Meet is developed by Google; another video communication service [39]. Usually, the unpaid subscription of meets limits up to 60 min duration and 100 users. The basic features of the meet are the multi-way audio–video encrypted call, integration with calendar and contacts, audio–video filtration, and augmented reality masks [40, 41].

Another software industry in line with the above is Microsoft which launched Teams for online teaching–learning and meetings [42–44]. It has replaced similar but two distinct products, i.e., Microsoft skype for business and Microsoft classroom. File sharing, group chat, calling, meeting, teaching, and live events are a few of the activities that can be accomplished with teams.

WebEx by Cisco is a cloud calling and screen sharing-based software launched to promote learning and professional preparation in today's digital age [45]. A web-hosted service named GoToMeeting was developed and marketed by LogMeIn in the year 2011 [46]. In this software, the data transmission is highly encrypted and optionally password-protected to enrich the security of users. Flipgrid [47–49] is an online software platform that equips learners for social interactions and discussions among students.

In addition to the above, there are some Android, iOS, macOS compatible applications, such as Canva, Padlet, G suite, Adobe spark, Book creator, and Anchor that somehow support online education, meeting, and discussion. Online assessment software packages, such as Google forms, Kami, Quizzes, Kahoot, EdPuzzle, and Gimkit are quite popular among the huge stack of similes.

Although all these recent software are suffering from a few bugs and security issues and will take a little more time to fix the same [50, 51]. Such issues are addressed and supported through the inclusion of online teaching–learning. The whole process of offline education system is transported into an online mode within a short span which is indeed incredible. However, a long way to go to make it more user-friendly and bug-free.

Digitization of Physical Documents

Digitization is the process to convert text, pictures, physical objects, and sound into a binary form so that they can be processed by computing devices. As compared to analog data, digital or binary data can easily be stored, processed, and shared with remote locations without or very fewer losses. Digitization is the prior step of digitalization to transport the business model on a digital platform.

Digitization process: Sampling and Quantization [52, 53]**:** The process of shortening a continuous analog signal into a discrete binary signal is known as Sampling or Discretization. The mapping of large set values into a smaller set is known as quantization. As shown below in Fig. 3.1, the black dots over the signal represent the sample points, whereas the horizontal dotted lines represent the quantization.

Various tools are available to convert physical documents into binary form. The scanner converts the images and documents into digital form for computer processing [54]. A 3D scanner transfers real-world objects' surfaces, such as hills, cars, human beings, etc., into discrete binary bit sequences [55]. A 3D scanning technology is used in image-sensor-equipped Digital cameras.

Digital pens are also used in this category to convert analog handwriting or drawing into a binary sequence [56]. However, Smartpen [57, 58] has a few more features, such as voice recording, text scanning, data storage, etc. In addition, digital pens are very useful for secondary students having learning disabilities [59]. Accelerometer, position, and camera-based digital pens are available in the market to capture analog data and digitize it.

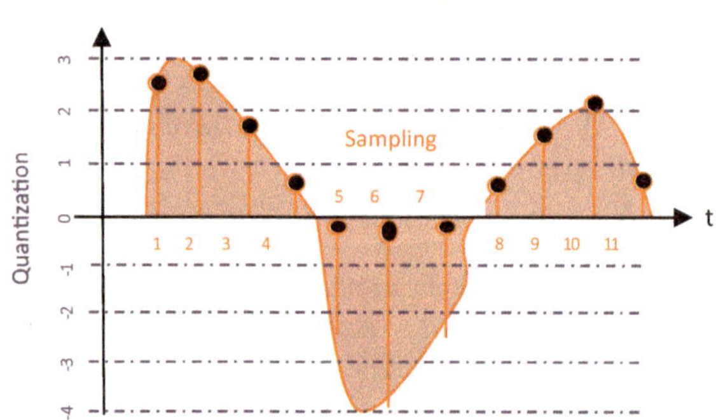

Fig. 3.1 Sampling and Quantization process of a continuous signal

Geographical Information System (GIS) converts any kind of data including geographical and Satellite rasters into an electronic map. It helps the user to understand the patterns and their relationship with geographical context for better control and decision-making [60, 61].

Sensors are one of the basic hardware requirements to digitize any physical object or document, and are thus used in the scanner, camera, and GIS-based hardware systems.

Digital Transformation: Developing Versus Developed Countries

The impact of digital reform can boost the economy, employability, and domestic productivity of a country. However, it is also true that the impact may vary between developing and developed countries in terms of required time and infrastructure complexity.

In developing countries, communication infrastructure is not well established so far, and thus the growth of digitization and digital reform is a little bit challenging. On the other hand, developed countries are well established in terms of communication technology and infrastructure, mobile and static electronic devices, and thus have better opportunities to spread digital transformation over existing foundations.

Developing Country: India

India is one of the fastest-growing economies in the Asia Pacific region and is rich in human resources as the second-largest populated country in the world. There is a scarcity of resources required for digital transformation in all the sections. Although the Government of India (GoI) offers opportunities to public and private sector companies, however, the resistance to change and the motivation level of students and teachers are the big hurdles in this domain.

The digital reform in the education sector needs to be carried forward systematically. Both, technology and digitized content are challenging issues in developing countries like India. An average speed of data communication and a smart device like a mobile, tablet, laptop, etc., are required to adapt to online education throughout the country and are not under the budget of a large population segment. Compared to developed countries, India is at least a generation behind in technical communication.

Digital gadgets: There are rural areas in India, where the issues of communications and smart devices exist in this era even. As per the study, only 42% of the Indian population have smartphones in the year 2020, and is expected to reach up to 51% by the year 2025. Around 11% of the population possess a computer that may be a desktop, laptop, notebook, netbook, palmtops, or tablet.

Internet usage: When it comes to internet usage, around only 50% of the population uses the internet. Indian telecom is one of the most competitive in the world with 11 wireless service providers. As per the data shared by Ookla's Speedtest Global Index, the average download speed of mobile devices in India is 12.41 Mbps and the upload speed is 4.76Mbps in January 2021, however, the average speed in a developed country is 25 Mbps.

In addition to the above issues, only 56% of rural schools have electricity, and 12% have functional computers as per the Indian government data. In due outbreak of Covid-19, the last two academic years are evaluated on pro-rata for primary, secondary, and higher secondary students [62]. Although, a few national and international level universities and institutes attempted to conduct the online examinations in proctored and non-proctored mode. However, the effort was not up to the mark as students have ways to escape academic integrity when not attempting in-person examination. An abrupt change in teaching–learning methodology causes a gap between students and teachers which is not good for the future perspective of the nation [63].

Though the challenges persist, the Indian government and associated educational bodies are taking the required measures and initiatives to enhance and incorporate digital technology in education, such as DIKSHA portal, e-Pathshala, Swayam, and STEM game-based education [64]. However, the quality of teachers, IT infrastructure, and awareness of digital technology are important parameters that need to be taken care of in the future.

Developed Country: USA

The developed countries, like the USA, have all the basic facilities, such as highways, electricity, technology, and communication infrastructure. Digitalization and digitization can easily be implemented over the existing infrastructure [65]. As per the USA government data, 100% of the population has been getting electricity since 1990.

They have well-equipped IoT-enabled smart cities, smart buildings, and classrooms. The internet download and upload speed is an average of around 25 Mbps throughout the country. Around 85% of the population uses smartphones in the USA. More than 90% of the population has digital devices, such as desktops, laptops, and tablets equipped with internet connectivity.

While developing countries are currently using 4G services and struggling to incorporate 5G, the USA has been using 5G since long ago. The teachers and students are well aware of digital technology in education. Very recently India has started to digitize the content and provide spaces for digital content for remote user access, whereas a lot of universities are running with electronic data utilization.

Enough resources are available in the developed countries and that is sufficient for digital reform in education [66]. However, artificial intelligence and expert system-based specialized hardware educational devices need to be explored shortly.

Chapter Conclusion and Future Urge

The impact and challenges of digital reform in education are different for developing and developed countries. The existing developed infrastructure and technological growth in terms of communication and digital gadgets are beneficial for digital reform in the education sector when it comes to developed countries. At the same time, developing countries are facing challenges in the adaptation, awareness, and technical training to the students, instructors, and guardians. In addition, to these issues, the availability of technical platforms both, software and hardware are not much mature to take care of in-person monitoring of students' growth.

The change in any established and well-working system is not possible overnight. Future opportunities in the digital education domain are:

(i) The teaching–learning pedagogy and monitoring of the examination process need to be strongly improvised.
(ii) COVID-19 pandemic accelerated digitization exponentially, and the utilization of technology and digital gadgets in education is highly expected and appreciated in the near future.
(iii) Government associates, as well as dedicated NGOs, need to honestly work on awareness drives among students, teachers, and guardians.
(iv) The available software platforms have some technical glitches. Although such glitches can be sorted out over time, more attentiveness is required while understanding the challenges and demands of teachers and students.

References

1. Moore, R.L., Fodrey B.P.: Distance education and technology infrastructure: strategies and opportunities. In: Leading and managing e-learning, pp. 87–100. Springer, Cham (2018)
2. Zhao, M., Liao, H-.T., Sun, S-.P.: An education literature review on digitization, digitalization, datafication, and digital transformation. In: 6th International Conference on Humanities and Social Science Research (ICHSSR 2020), pp. 302–306. Atlantis Press (2020)
3. Karakozov, S.D., Ryzhova, N.I.: Information and education systems in the context of digitalization of education. J. Sib. Fed. Univ.: Hum.Ities Soc. Sci. **12**(9), 1635–1647 (2019)
4. Mertala, P.: Paradoxes of participation in the digitalization of education: a narrative account. Learn. Media Technol. **45**(2), 179–192 (2020)
5. Machekhina, O.N.: Digitalization of education as a trend of its modernization and reforming. Revista Espacios **38**(40) (2017)
6. Lubkov, A.V., Gordienko, O.V., Sokolova, A.A.: A humanitarian approach to the digitization of education. Educ. Self Dev. 89–96 (2020)
7. Perry, C.A.: Education for digitization: how do we prepare? J. Acad. Librariansh. **31**(6), 523–532 (2005)
8. Telukdarie, A., Munsamy, M.: Digitization of Higher Education Institutions. In: 2019 IEEE International Conference on Industrial Engineering and Engineering Management (IEEM), pp. 716–721. IEEE (2019)
9. Strokov, A.A.: Digitalization of education: problems and prospects. Vestn. Minin Univ. **2**(31) pp. 15 (2020)

10. Bejinaru, R.: Impact of digitalization on education in the knowledge economy. Manag. Dyn. Knowl. Econ. **7**(3), 367–380 (2019)
11. Vlieghe, J.: Education, digitization and literacy training: a historical and cross-cultural perspective. Educ. Philos. Theory **48**(6), 549–562 (2016)
12. Anju, P., Sharma, H.L.: Effectiveness of EDUCOMP smart classroom teaching on achievement in mathematics at elementary level. IJAR **2**(6), 683–687 (2016)
13. Balihara, A., Venkatesh, G.: A Study on Rapid Growth of Educomp Solutions Limited (2011)
14. Alturki, U.T., Aldraiweesh, A.: Evaluating the usability and accessibility of LMS "Blackboard" at King Saud University. Contemp. Issues Educ. Res. (CIER) **9**(1), 33–44 (2016)
15. Tawalbeh, T.I.: EFL instructors' perceptions of blackboard learning management system (LMS) at University level. Engl. Lang. Teach. **11**(1), 1–9 (2018)
16. Subramanian, P., Zainuddin, N., Alatawi, S., Javabdeh, T., Hussin, A.: A study of comparison between Moodle and Blackboard based on case studies for better LMS. J. Inf. Syst. Res. Innov. **6**, 26–33 (2014)
17. K. Al-Omar: Evaluating the usability and learnability of the "blackboard" LMS using SUS and data mining. In: 2018 Second International Conference on Computing Methodologies and Communication (ICCMC), pp. 386–390 (2018). https://doi.org/10.1109/ICCMC.2018.8488038
18. Cole, J., Foster, H.: Using Moodle: Teaching with the Popular Open Source Course Management System. O'Reilly Media, Inc (2007)
19. Lu, J., Law, N.W.Y.: Understanding collaborative learning behavior from Moodle log data. Interact. Learn. Environ. **20**(5), 451–466 (2012)
20. Wu, W.-S., Hua, C.: The application of Moodle on an EFL collegiate writing environment. J. Educ. Foreign Lang. Lit. **7**(1), 45–56 (2008)
21. Tsai, Y.-R., Talley, P.C.: The effect of a course management system (CMS)-supported strategy instruction on EFL reading comprehension and strategy use. Comput. Assist. Lang. Learn. **27**(5), 422–438 (2014)
22. Cerezo, R., Sánchez-Santillán, M., Puerto Paule-Ruiz, M., Carlos Núñez, J.: Students' LMS interaction patterns and their relationship with achievement: a case study in higher education. Comput. Educ. **96**, 42–54 (2016)
23. Rabiman, R., Nurtanto, M., Kholifah, N.: Design and development E-learning system by learning management system (LMS) in vocational education. Online Submission **9**(1), 1059–1063 (2020)
24. Villegas-Ch, W., Román-Cañizares,M., Palacios-Pacheco, X.: Improvement of an online education model with the integration of machine learning and data analysis in an LMS. Appl. Sci. **10**(15), 5371 (2020)
25. Chassignol, M., Khoroshavin, A., Klimova, A., Bilyatdinova, A.: Artificial intelligence trends in education: a narrative overview. Proc. Comput. Sci. **136**, 16–24 (2018)
26. Kavitha, V., Lohani, R.: A critical study on the use of artificial intelligence, e-Learning technology and tools to enhance the learners experience. Clust. Comput. **22**(3), 6985–6989 (2019)
27. Waks, L.J.: MOOCs and career qualifications. In: The Evolution and Evaluation of Massive Open Online Courses, pp. 83–101. Palgrave Pivot, New York (2016)
28. Kolowich, S.: How EdX plans to earn, and share, revenue from its free online courses. Chron. High. Educ. **21** (2013)
29. Kumar, A., Agrawal, A., Agrawal, P.: Massive open online courses: EdX. org, Coursera. com and NPTEL, a comparative study based on usage statistics and features with special reference to India (2015)
30. Young, J.R.: Inside the Coursera contract: How an upstart company might profit from free courses. Chron. High. Educ. **19**(07) (2012)
31. Bates, T.: What's right and what's wrong about Coursera-style MOOCs. EdTech in the Wild (2019)
32. ur Rehman, I., Bano, S., Mehraj, M..: MOOCS: A case study of ALISON platform. Libr. Philos. Pract. 1–8 (2019)

33. Sheeja, Nk.: Open educational resources in India: a study of NPTEL and its usage." Libr. Her. **56**(1), 122–129 (2018)
34. Busteed, B.: Why Goodwill (Not Udacity, edX or Coursera) may be the World's biggest MOOC. Forbes **26** (2019)
35. Oktavia, T., Prabowo, H., Supangkat, S.H.: The comparison of MOOC (massive open online course) platforms of edx and coursera (study case: student of programming courses). In: 2018 International Conference on Information Management and Technology (ICIMTech), pp. 339–344. IEEE (2018)
36. Singh, R., Awasthi, S.: Updated comparative analysis on video conferencing platforms-Zoom, Google Meet, Microsoft Teams, WebEx Teams and GoToMeetings. EasyChair: The World for Scientists, pp. 1–9 (2020)
37. Zhang, X., Chen, Q., Ren Ng, Koltun, V.: Zoom to learn, learn to zoom. In: Proceedings of the IEEE/CVF Conference on Computer Vision and Pattern Recognition, pp. 3762–3770 (2019)
38. Mohanty, M., Yaqub, W.: Towards seamless authentication for Zoom-based online teaching and meeting (2020). arXiv preprint arXiv:2005.10553
39. Perez, S.: Google quietly launches Meet, an enterprise-friendly version of Hangouts. TechCrunch. AOL. Archived from the original Retrieved (2017)
40. Nasution, A.R., Nandiyanto, A.B.D.: Utilization of the google meet and quiziz applications in the assistance and strengthening process of online learning during the COVID-19 pandemic. Indones. J. Educ. Res. Technol. **1**(1), 31–34 (2021)
41. Sette-de-Souza, P.H.: Motivating learners in pandemic period through WhatsApp and Google Meet. J. Dent. Educ. (2020)
42. Hubbard, M., Bailey, M.J.: Mastering Microsoft Teams. Mastering Microsoft Teams. https://doi.org/10.1007/978-1-4842-3670-3 (2018)
43. Ilag, B.N.: Microsoft Teams overview. In: Understanding Microsoft Teams Administration, pp. 1–36. Apress, Berkeley, CA (2020)
44. Pal, D., Vanijja, V.: Perceived usability evaluation of Microsoft Teams as an online learning platform during COVID-19 using system usability scale and technology acceptance model in India. Child Youth Serv. Rev. **119**, 105535 (2020)
45. WebEx, Cisco: Why WebEx." Connect with anyone, anywhere, anytime. http://www.webex.com/why-webex/overview.html (2014). Retrieved 12 Dec 2012
46. Perron, B., Ruffolo, M.: A review of a web-conferencing technology. GoTo meeting (2011)
47. Green, T., Green, J.: Flipgrid: Adding voice and video to online discussions. TechTrends **62**(1), 128–130 (2018)
48. Bartlett, M.: Using Flipgrid to increase students' connectedness in an online class. eLearn , (12) (2018)
49. Keiper, M.C., White, A., Carlson, C.D., Lupinek, J.M.: Student perceptions on the benefits of Flipgrid in a HyFlex learning environment. J. Educ. Bus. 1–9 (2020)
50. John, A.St.: It's Not Just Zoom. Google Meet, Microsoft Teams, and Webex Have Privacy Issues, Too (2020)
51. Gauthier, N.H., Husain, M.I.: Dynamic security analysis of Zoom, Google Meet and Microsoft Teams. In: Silicon Valley Cybersecurity Conference: First Conference, SVCC 2020, San Jose, CA, USA, December 17–19, 2020, Revised Selected Papers, vol. 1383, p. 3. Springer Nature (2021)
52. Santina, M.S., Stubberud, A.R.: Basics of sampling and quantization. In: Handbook of networked and embedded control systems, pp. 45–69. Birkhäuser Boston (2005)
53. Johansson, H.: Sampling and quantization. In: Academic Press Library in Signal Processing, vol. 1, pp. 169–244. Elsevier (2014)
54. Safonov, I.V., Kurilin, I.V., Rychagov, M.N., Tolstaya, E.V.: Document Image Processing for Scanning and Printing. Springer (2019)
55. Daneshmand, M., Helmi, A., Avots, E., Noroozi, F., Alisinanoglu, F., Arslan, H.S., Gorbova, J., Haamer, R.E., Ozcinar, C., Anbarjafari, G.: 3D scanning: a comprehensive survey (2018). arXiv preprint arXiv:1801.08863

56. Schreiner, K.: Uniting the paper and digital worlds. IEEE Comput. Graphics Appl. **28**(6), 6–10 (2008)
57. Uskov, V.L., Howlett, R.J., Jain, L.C. (eds.) Smart Education and Smart E-Learning, vol. 41. Springer (2015)
58. Tucker, L., Zamfir, B.: Student perception on the impact of the Livescribe smartpen as an accommodation. Univers. Access Inf. Soc. 1–9 (2021)
59. Ok, M.W., Rao, K.: Using a digital pen to support secondary students with learning disabilities. Interv. Sch. Clin. **53**(1), 36–43 (2017)
60. Raju, P.L.N.: Fundamentals of geographical information system. Satellite Remote Sensing and GIS Applications in Agricultural Meteorology, vol. 103 (2006)
61. Wiegand, P.: Geographical information systems (GIS) in education. Interv. Sch. Clin. **10**(1), 68–71 (2001)
62. Maity, S., Sahu, T.N., Sen, N.: Panoramic view of digital education in COVID-19: A new explored avenue. Rev. Educ. **9**(2), 405–423 (2021)
63. Iivari, N., Sharma, S., Ventä-Olkkonen, L.: Digital transformation of everyday life–How COVID-19 pandemic transformed the basic education of the young generation and why information management research should care? Int. J. Inf. Manage. **55**, 102183 (2020)
64. Singh, M., Adebayo, S.O., Saini, M., Singh, J.: Indian government E-learning initiatives in response to COVID-19 crisis: a case study on online learning in Indian higher education system. Educ. Inf. Technol. 1–39 (2021)
65. Pramanik, H.S., Kirtania, M., Pani, A.K.: Essence of digital transformation—Manifestations at large financial institutions from North America. Futur. Gener. Comput. Syst. **95** 323–343 (2019)
66. Kutnjak, A., Pihiri, I., Furjan, M.T.: Digital transformation case studies across industries—literature review. In: 2019 42nd International Convention on Information and Communication Technology, Electronics and Microelectronics (MIPRO), pp. 1293–1298. https://doi.org/10.23919/MIPRO.2019.8756911 (2019)

Chapter 4
Digitalization of Education—Challenges and Measures for Promotion

Anuradha Chavali and Vijayalaxmi Biradar

Introduction

If online reports are to be believed, by the close of 2025, there would be an increase in the internet penetration rate by more than 55% in India. Covid-19 has caused a major setback to conventional education and has paved the way for digitalisation of education being the immediate priority for the Indian Government. Academic institutions, digital companies and e-learning portals to name a few have been quick enough to respond to the changes in the post-pandemic scenario. E-learning portals have come up with diverse online courses, universities are busy designing more comprehensive online degree, diploma and specialisation programmes offered worldwide. Given the opportunity, there has been substantial growth in the Ed-Tech companies catering to the need for learning management resources-incorporating technology into learning using algorithms based on artificial intelligence, turning blending learning into reality, providing 3D and DIY kits to name a few, integrated to offer an unparalleled pragmatic and interactive teaching–learning experience.

Traditional Education

The main impetus in conventional education back then was on schools as formal means of education and community libraries or so when it came to informal education. The mode of delivery was the lecture method in the classroom with textbooks

A. Chavali
Department of Business Administration, ICFAI University, Hyderabad, India

V. Biradar (✉)
Department of Electrical & Electronics Engineering, Kalinga University, Raipur, India
e-mail: dr.vijayalaxmi@kalingauniversity.ac.in

A. Choudhury et al. (eds.), *Evolution of Digitized Societies Through Advanced Technologies*, Advanced Technologies and Societal Change,
https://doi.org/10.1007/978-981-19-2984-7_4

and notes that were prepared from the knowledge and experiences of the teachers over time, being the reference material for learning. The students had to seek admission into the formal academic institutions and physically attend the classes to finish their formal education. Institute libraries provided them with further references. The instructor or the teacher had to be an epitome of knowledge on one hand and proficient in delivering the same without losing the attention of the students on the other. Hence, not only knowledge acquisition, but transferring the same and ensuring retention by the student was equally important for a teacher.

But with time, there has been a paradigm shift in the nature and scope of education.

Digital Learning

The year 1999 saw the beginning of what we call digital learning when it was propounded by Jay Cross [1]. Advancements in technology from time to time have added to new terms and theories pertaining to it. As has been underlined by Doris Holzberger et al. (2013), e-learning can be attributed to the dissemination of education through the internet with the objective of elevating knowledge acquisition and retention along with developing design skills.

It was all about using computers and networking in creating learning environments so as to get over the limitations of geographical boundaries and time, and to make it more learner-centric and alter it in a way that allows for individualised learning [2].

As is propounded by the American Society of Training and Education (ASTD), digital learning is the application of digital media to the field of learning with the coming together of the network service providers and the required hardware and the software applications all resulting in computer-based learning and evaluation across the networks in virtual class spaces.

According to Anttila et al. [3], e-learning is used as a contrivance for accessing learning material. There are numerous definitions put across to explain digital learning across the globe. A close analysis of the same would help us to classify it into four quadrants in line with the observations of Keane, 2012:

1. Access to teaching–learning material in the form of digital books
2. Usage of digital tools
3. Delivery medium
4. Independent learning

Bidding farewell to the conventional teaching techniques and shortcomings like the scarcity of qualified workforce, insufficient student–teacher ratio, non-availability of adequate resources, digitalisation has paved way for novel approaches in learning with the objective of increasing accessibility and improving technology usage skills for both the educators and the learners, thus contributing to individual and societal goals.

The Impact of Digital Learning

Undoubtedly, technology has come to the rescue of the educational sector that has been hard hit by the onset of Covid-19. Even as the country is moving towards plans to get back to physical campus learning, the importance of technology in education should not be undermined. Though imbibing technology with education presents a rosy optimistic picture of facilitating personalised and specialised learning, economical in terms of time, effort and money and empowering the young people with digital skills that would contribute to the needs of the corporate world of the years to come, but one should not be carried away to an extent that we do not look at the larger side of the picture.

Let us start with a question, will digital learning continue to contribute even after the restoration of normalcy, and what is going to look like? What would be the role of ICT in the classroom and beyond? How would the technology be blended to provide a learning experience that would be effective in terms of extent and intensity along with the pedagogy?

One should not get carried away by the merits of digitalization of education that they fail to see the other side of technology and its link with the student outcomes, given the internal and external factors in our country:

The device type that is used may sometimes result in the most awful outcomes.

- The geographical location is one of the determinants of outcome with rural areas exhibiting poor outcomes
- The intensity with which it is used may also have an effect on the outcome
- The philosophy, the climate and the culture of the institution also effects on the student performance.

These issues need to be conceptually framed and empirically tested to develop a system that would help us to harvest the benefit of integration of technology with education.

Leading Concerns About the Future of Digital Learning

The pandemic presents innumerable intimidations to education and all the parties affected by it, be it the instructors, institutions, students or parents. The much talked about the risk associated with the digital learning is how well is our country given its widespread digital divide is ready to go ahead with mighty technological platforms with up to date digital content, engagement of the educators coupled with the vision and commitment of the private management of the educational institutions and the Government in improving the same.

What cannot be denied is the lack of infrastructural and procedural facilities that would support digitalisation of education in our country and the challenges faced in these turbulent times battered by ground realities and inequalities making the transition all the more difficult.

Another matter of concern is the reliance of the educational institutions on their own faculty members for the preparation of digital content instead of approaching agencies with experience in preparing such content.

Added to the list is the risk as to how the technology providers would respond to the new set of needs arising out of digitalisation. Michael Feldstein enunciates the concern appropriately in his explanation of the billion-dollar ed-tech hole. According to Michael Feldstein, vendors try to provide solutions as per the specifications of the customers but what remains a challenge is the area the customers are really aware of what they need? In the absence of this clarity, vendors tend to deliver what appears to be solutions, but actually, they aggravate the problem.

Digital learning in India is not a problem of the policy makers or the Government. It is something that is interrelated and interdependent on all the subsystems of acquisition, adherence to quality, answerability, evaluation and assessment and so on of a greater ecosystem. For instance:

- Do we have adequate funds for preparation and implementation of digital content?
- Is a suitable professional help and facilitation being provided to the educators?
- How successfully can we blend the digital content and assessment into the formal learning and bring it to the mainstream?
- What is the contribution of educational technology service providers' role?
- What is the extent of awareness about the existing modules and their efficacies?

Ironically, all these questions have been addressed in varied ways and most of the times erroneously given the inadequate planning in this direction. This results in faulty policies and implementation, thus defeating the entire purpose of digitalisation. The ideal elucidation to battle this limitation is to align our educational goals with these questions and seek appropriate solutions, given the internal and external constraints.

With the dawn of digital education, our primary question was how was it going to contribute to learning but now Covid-19 has made it an inevitable option and everyone is looking eagerly as to how digital education would come to our rescue, the goals that it would support and the roadmap for its implementation.

As of now, the educational sector is going through a crisis and it needs immediate intervention by responding to the immediate challenges posed by the pandemic that would have long term implications for the individuals, organisations and the society at large.

Once we objectively evaluate these questions and normalcy is restored, the entire ecosystem would seek answers to the questions as to

- What is that we are trying to achieve in the days to come?
- How would we go about it so as to have benefits that would be everlasting?

One needs to seek answers to these inevitable questions as decisions which would have a profound impact upon the education sector and all the stakeholders affected by it have to be taken. Right now with the need for digitalisation of education, the policy makers are arriving at decisions as to what would result in a long heave but the implications of the decisions are yet to be clear.

Supporting Technologies and Its Applications

The education sector in India is passing through a wave of digitalisation, thanks to the technological improvements which have introduced high end gadgets, novel innovative training tools and modern state-of-the-art equipment, all contributing to creation and dissemination of knowledge like never before.

Virtual Reality (VR)

Virtual Reality (VR) as the name suggests employs VR headsets in combination of various props and environments to create sounds and images that replicate the reality and help the user experience a physical presence in a virtual environment.

The scope of VR has been extended beyond gaming and has been imbibed in the areas of learning and training as well as in music, sports and films.

Augmented Reality (AR)

Augmented Reality has complemented digital learning by making it more attractive to have more learner retention by providing them with an experience of what is being taught by superimposing computer generated content with the real world by using graphics, sounds and videos.

Artificial Intelligence (AI)

This is something that has transformed the entire digital learning by helping the learners to identify their areas of improvement with cutting-edge AI models solving complex problems in an inclusive way as compared to the conventional classrooms.

Big Data

Big Data facilitates the preparation of learning modules and interactions between the users and monitors the learning patterns, based on which one understands where the learners struggle or excel and this acts as input to improve upon the modules to provide the learners with unsurpassed outcomes.

Machine Learning

This is a solution for tailor fit learning that would precisely provide the resources needed and would align with the past performance of the learner and the goals to be attained.

Wearable Devices

Wearables are compact but smart electronic devices when worn on the body are capable of taking scenarios and simulations over and beyond expectations and make learning all the more interesting and intelligible.

The deployment of all the above technologies can really bring about notable changes in e-learning in India with unparalleled experiences not only to the students, but also to the educators. The ed-tech firms need to bank upon the development of such technologies and should upgrade themselves continuously to avoid the risk of becoming obsolete. Optimum utilisation of all the existing resources, using their strengths to make use of the opportunity available should be the objective of such firms, thereby providing the country with better learning outcomes.

There are scores of Apps and e-learning tools in the higher education sector that are primarily free but one can upgrade for better enrichment at a nominal cost not only for the student community, but also for the educators (Table 4.1).

Table 4.1 Scores of Apps and e-learning tools in higher education

Recording/collecting	Management	Security	Knowledge building
Office Lens Notability Dragon Microphone SoundNote	Uni Calculator iStudiez SimpleMind SelfControl StudyBlue GoConqr My Study Life **Timetable** EasyBib Google Drive Pinterest Coursera Google Duo Monzo	bSafe Circle Of 6	TED Talks Behance Duolingo Dictionary.com Exam Vocabulary Builder

List of Free e-Learning Platforms Developed by the Government of India

- **Swayam:** The Government of India has come up with SWAYAM that hosts diverse courses from 9th grade onwards till post-graduation with an objective of providing a mechanism for learning for all, even the most underprivileged.
- **Diksha:** It is yet another initiative by the Ministry of Education where the educators and the learners can access various courses in line with the CBSE, NCERT and SCERT nationwide.
- **e-ShodhSindhu:** This provides an access to more than 10,000 current as well as archived peer reviewed journals and numerous databases—bibliographic, citation and factual for its member institutions
- **e-PG Pathshala:** This is yet another meticulous effort by the MHRD in line with the National Mission on Education through ICT, and is being implemented by UGC with interactive digital content across 70 or more faculties of social sciences, arts, fine arts, natural and mathematical sciences.
- **Swayam Prabha:** It provides high precision educational content across the clock with 34 DTH dedicated channels with the content prepared by the IITs, NCERT, IGNOU, NIOS and so on.
- **NPTEL:** The National Programme on Technology Enhanced Learning is a remarkable initiative for providing open online courses in engineering and allied disciplines and is initiated by the IITs across the country in association with IISC, Bangalore.

Challenges

What remains a challenge is to break the existing way of knowledge acquisition and transfer and assimilation of digital technologies in education, not to forget the adaptation of the same by the teachers and the learners within a precise academic framework so as to eliminate vagueness in learning. In any attempt to do so, one would come across an outcome gap between anticipations and reality, when it comes to adopting a new approach both in theory and practice. A closer look at these so-called obstacles would help us to categorise them into explicit factors and implicit factors.

The external explicit factors act as the primary barriers. In line with the theory of Ertmer et al., 2012, one can categorise them into:

(1) Reach
(2) Organisational Factors
(3) Content
(4) Formative and Summative Assessment

The most important influence here is the fact that the instructors, as well as the learners, should be able to access the same. The popularity of digital technology in education is only possible if the parties to it can reach the necessary hardware, software and infrastructural provision and facilitation [4]. Added to it is the constant upgradation of technology that requires the parties to constantly upgrade themselves with the changes, which in itself is a meticulous task [5].

As is believed by [4], The academic institutions act as change agents here by developing an appropriate climate and culture that would facilitate the absorption of technology in education and strong leadership that would translate the need for the same for all the stakeholders so as to turn the resistance to change into acceptance. A lot needs to be done in terms of bringing about awareness, removing fears and apprehensions, providing necessary support and facilitation, increasing the morale and motivation, and above all, giving the time break to internalise and adapt to the changes.

The perception of the educators and the learner community about the types of digital tutoring has an effect on the workability of digitalisation, and so is the response of the institutions towards innovation (Ertmer et al., 2012. The curriculum that needs to fit into the framework and the need for objective assessment also pose a challenge to digital education [4],6]. What is needed in India is a transition from conventional learning to digitalisation where educators use digital technology and align their pedagogy for achieving positive student outcomes. But there are influences from the other social-cultural elements which cannot be ignored [7–9].

Whenever there are any changes introduced in the subsystems, they may have a domino effect within the system and the same is true in case of digitalisation of education. There is a lot of resistance, and if it is not handled adequately, it may make it difficult to be implemented and would affect the overall efficacy of learning [9, 10].

Along with the external influences, the practices that are followed by the educators comprises the internal influence and act as a barrier of second order and make integration and implementation of technology difficult (Ertmer et al., 2007, Blackwell et al., 2013) [11, 25].

The true doorkeepers are the implicit factors that exert conflict within the individual, whether it be a student or a teacher or any other stakeholder (Ertmer et al., 2012). These can be enlisted as the beliefs and the predispositions of the people, the conventional models and the need to break the stereotypes, the diverse skills and the knowledge required and redesign and reengineering of the organisations and the need to align academics to tailor fit them to the requirements of the corporate world. The attitude makes all the difference, be it of the teachers or the students, as it affects the acceptance or resistance towards digital learning and engagement with the same [11] (Pegler et al., 2010).

As has been advocated by Cranton and King (2003) [12], the personal attitudes, value systems and beliefs and norms affect the professional functioning as well and have an effect on the practices in the organisation [11] (Pegler et al., 2010; Petko, 2012). The educators who believe in teacher-centric learning may resist the digitalisation of education which is more student-centric (Ertmer and Ottenbreit-Leftwich, 2010) [13]. The same is the case with routines that form a major goal in the conventional education model and a practice that is considered to be inherently important but the same is disturbed when we go for digital integration [14].

A diverse range of internal and external factors make the process of integration and the realisation of the benefits of digital education a complex process. Though there has been an elevation in the reach and adoption of technological advancements, still they are not in line with the expectations [15]. Hence, there is still a lot of ambiguity and uncertainty and many questions and apprehensions unanswered [6]. The management of this transition is a slow and complex one. The very assumption of digital learning may contradict the teacher and student's perception of its viability, thus making it difficult to incorporate into the conventional system. Added to it is the fact that the pedagogies that are developed by amalgamation of various technologies and platforms are still not widely understood and accepted. Similarly, there is a dearth of promotion of the same and attempts to clear the apprehensions of all the stakeholders [16]. The need for incorporating technology in the education sector has been accelerated due to the advent of Covid-19, but still there is a lot to be done in the direction of developing metrics for measuring its success. One can find the explicit influences of digital technologies, but it is still a bigger challenge to define the implicit influences and provide a framework for conceptualising the interplay between the explicit and implicit influences.

Conclusion

One cannot ignore the contribution of education to economic growth and development. The rolling out of the New Education Policy, 2020, is a clear indication of the importance that is attached to the digitalisation of education in promoting continuous student-centric learning. Paramount attention has been garnered towards the rural areas by making education accessible to all the nooks and corners of the country, especially the 2- and 3-tier towns and villages. What was impossible earlier can be realised with the integration of technology with education. As is evident from the Budget 2021–22, ₹93,224.31 crores have been allocated to the Ministry of Education which is almost a ₹8,100 crore increase.

The hue and cry over the transition towards digitalisation of education have garnered attention towards the huge digital divide prevalent in India and the need for readiness from all the stakeholders, each representing a different set of challenges towards the preparedness for the same. When it comes to schools, this divide is visibly high as compared to higher education institutions. There is a lot to be done to bridge the gap whether in terms of urban and rural areas, government and private institutions or schools and higher education institutions. Digital accessibility and reach need to be improved across the institutions no matter whatever the geographical location, financial condition and infrastructural amenities available so far.

Formative and summative assessment needs to be aligned with the new trends of digital education facilitating custom made exercises, online proctoring and ratification and certification besides providing a secure, reliable and credible platform that is economical in terms of time, effort and money by saving on operational, personnel, organisational and logistics driven costs.

Suitable procedural and policy changes need to be brought about not only in creating infrastructure, but also in terms of talent acquisition, curriculum development and evaluation and assessment metrics. If the country is successful in taking proactive measures and suitable interventions, there would be a huge paradigm shift in the education sector of India with the most evolving technologies suitable for the education sector in place, thereby revamping the digital fabric of the country and providing it with a global competitive advantage. Digital and e-learning are undoubtedly the future and the ed-tech companies that need to partner with this change and cater to the needs of digitalisation of education.

There would be a drastic change in the teaching–learning process in the years to come with the adoption of digital mode not only in the lines of admittance, access and transfer, but also assessment of learning that would become the new normal post the pandemic. All this would lead to a paradigm shift in the digitally powered academic arena with numerous opportunities for youth leading to an empowered India.

References

1. Yoon, J., Kwon, S., Shim, J.E.: Present status and issues of school nutrition programs in Korea. Asia Pac. J. Clin. Nutr. **21**(1), 128–133 (2012)
2. Kaklamanou, D., Pearce, J., Nelson, M.: (2012). Food and Academies: A Qualitative Study. Department for Education, pp. 1–23
3. Anttila, M., Valimaki, M., Hatonen, H., Luukkaala, T., Kaila, M.: Use of web-based patient education sessions on psychiatric wards. Int. J. Med. Informatics **81**(6), 424–433 (2012)
4. Fu, J.S.: ICT in education: a critical literature review and its implications. Int. J. Educ. Dev. Using Inf. Commun. Technol. **9**(1), 112–125 (2013)
5. Skues, J.L., Cunningham, E.G.: The role of e-learning coaches in Australian secondary schools. J. Comput. Assist. Learn. **29**(2), 179–187 (2013). https://doi.org/10.1111/j.1365-2729.2012.00488.x
6. Orlando, J.: ICT-mediated practice and constructivist practices: Is this still the best plan for teachers' uses of ICT? Technol. Pedagog. Educ. **22**(2), 231–246 (2013). https://doi.org/10.1080/1475939X.2013.782702
7. Feldman, A., Weiss, T.: Understanding change in teachers' ways of being through collaborative action research: a cultural–historical activity theory analysis. Educ. Action Res. **18**(1), 29–55 (2010). https://doi.org/10.1080/09650790903484517
8. Nielsen, W., Miller, A., Hoban, G.F.: The digital education revolution: New South Wales science teachers' response to laptop ubiquity. AERA Annual Meeting 2012. Retrieved from http://ro.uow.edu.au/edupapers/1086/ (2012)
9. Tay, L.Y., Lim, S.K., Lim, C.P.: Factors affecting the ICT integration and implementation of one-to-one computing learning environment in a primary school—A sociocultural perspective. In: Tay, L.Y., Lim, C.P. (eds.) Tales from a future school in Singapore, pp. 19–37. Sense Publishers, Rotterdam (2013)
10. Engeström, Y.: Expansive learning: toward an activity-theoretical reconceptualization. In: Illeris, K. (ed.) Contemporary Theories Of Learning: Learning Theorists in Their Own Words. Routledge, New York (2009a)

11. Hsu, S., Kuan, P.-Y.: The impact of multilevel factors on technology integration: the case of Taiwanese grade 1–9 teachers and schools. Educ. Tech. Res. Dev. **61**(1), 25–50 (2013). https://doi.org/10.1007/s11423-012-9269-y
12. Galvis, H.A.: Understanding beliefs, teachers' beliefs and their impact on the use of computer technology. PROFILE **14**(2), 95–112 (2012)
13. Mama, M., Hennessy, S.: Developing a typology of teacher beliefs and practices concerning classroom use of ICT. Comput. Educ. **68**, 380–387 (2013). https://doi.org/10.1016/j.compedu.2013.05.022
14. Somekh, B.: Pedagogy and learning with ICT: Researching the art of innovation [Kindleversion]. Retrieved from http://www.amazon.com/dp/B001QMT6MO/ref=r_soa_w_d (2007)
15. Howard, S.K., Mozejko, A.: Considering the history of digital technologies in education. In: Henderson, M., Romero, G. (eds.) Teaching and Digital Technologies: Big Issues and Critical Questions, pp. 157–168. Cambridge University Press, Port Melbourne, Australia (2015)
16. Fullan, M.: Stratosphere—Integrating Technology, Pedagogy, and Change Knowledge. Pearson, Toronto (2013)
17. ACARA: Information and communication technology (ICT) capability. Retrieved March, 2016, from Australian Curriculum, Assessment and Reporting Authority http://www.australiancurriculum.edu.au/generalcapabilities/information-and-communicationtechnology-capability/introduction/introduction (2014)
18. Engeström, Y., Sannino, A.: Studies of expansive learning: foundations, findings and future challenges. Educ. Res. Rev. **5**(1), 1–24 (2010). https://doi.org/10.1016/j.edurev.2009.12.002
19. Ertmer, P.A., Ottenbreit-Leftwich, A.: Removing obstacles to the pedagogical changes required by Jonassen's vision of authentic technology-enabled learning. Computers Education **64**, 175–182 (2013). https://doi.org/10.1016/j.compedu.2012.10.00
20. Harris, J., Hofer, M.: Learning Activity Types Wiki. Retrieved from http://activitytypes.wmwikis.net/HOME (2011)
21. Wastiau, P., Blamire, R., Kearney, C., Quittre, V., Van de Gaer, E., Monseur, C.: The use of ICT in education: a survey of schools in Europe. Eur. J. Educ. **48**, 11–27 (2013). https://doi.org/10.1111/ejed.12020
22. Koehler, M., Mishra, P.: What is technological pedagogical content knowledge (TPACK)? Contemp. Issues Technol. Teach. Educ. **9**(1), 60–70 (2009)
23. McKiernan, G.: Configuring the 'Future Textbook.' Search **19**(4), 43–47 (2011)
24. Miyoshi, M., Tsuboyama-Kasaoka, N.: School-based "Shokuiku" program in Japan: application to nutrition education in Asian countries. Asia Pac. J. Clin. Nutr. **21**(1), 159–162 (2012)
25. Vanderlinde, R., van Braak, J.: The e-capacity of primary schools: development of a conceptual model and scale construction from a school improvement perspective. Comput. Educ. **53**, 5410553 (2010). https://doi.org/10.1016/j.compedu.2010.02.016
26. "Get Ready to Hear a Lot More About 'XR'". Wired 1 May 2019. ISSN 1059-1028. Retrieved 29 Aug 2020
27. Psotka, J.: Immersive training systems: virtual reality and education and training. Instr. Sci. **23**(5), 405–431 (1995). https://doi.org/10.1007/BF00896880.S2CID60705937
28. "Online Etymology Dictionary".
29. Artaud, A.: The Theatre and its Double Trans. Mary Caroline Richards. Grove Weidenfeld, New York (1958)
30. Faisal, A.: "Computer science: visionary of virtual reality. Nature **551**(7680), 298–299 (2017). Bibcode: 2017Natur.551.298F. https://doi.org/10.1038/551298a
31. The definition of cyberspace.
32. Schnipper, M.: Seeing is Believing: The State of Virtual Reality. The Verge. Retrieved 7 March 2017
33. Baltrušaitis, J., Strachan, W.J.:. Anamorphic Art, p. 4.. Harry N. Abrams, New York (1977). ISBN 9780810906624

34. Brockwell, H.: Forgotten genius: the man who made a working VR machine in 1957. Tech Radar (2016). Retrieved 7 March 2017
35. "National Center for Supercomputing Applications: History". The Board of Trustees of the University of Illinois. Archived 21 Aug 2015

Chapter 5
Of Pandemic and Pedagogic Reconstruction: An Epistemological Enquiry into Digital Education in India

Debanjali Roy

Digital Domain and Changing Classrooms

With unprecedented technological advancements in the last few decades, there has been a global surge to harness digital potential in previously uncharted quarters like the domain of education. Burgeoning digital technology and more specifically, the internet, initiated the foraging of technology in classrooms, altering the essential fabric of education, noticeably. Triggered by this integration, the need for scrutinizing hitherto existing learning theories was recognized as was the necessity envisaged for accommodating the techno-space in the teaching–learning milieu. This has led to revisions in classroom pedagogy, pedagogic principles, and the concept of classroom itself, in recent times. A major revision has been the reconceptualization of "classrooms" where digitally conceptualized classrooms debunk the traditional idea of a fixed site for learning by envisioning a metamorphosis of the spatio-temporal infrastructure into a techno-space. In the Foreword to *Conceptualising the Digital University: The Intersection of Policy, Pedagogy and Practice*, Prof. Darder calls it the "Fourth Industrial Revolution" and connects this technological proliferation with an aggressive twist of old neoliberal values by economic deterministic rhetoric [1, p. x]. Referring to the twenty-first century as "the Knowledge Age", owing to the attachment of socio-economic values to knowledge and education, Linda Harasim rightly argues that "in our technology-driven world, it is critical and timely to study the intersection of learning theory and technology" [2, p. 2]. However, besides understanding the capacity of technology to reconfigure the educational paradigm, it is important to realize that "educational change and innovation, especially with technology, can be very complex, contingent on many different actors and factors" (Heppell, 2016 cited in Hall [3, p. 25]). The challenge to envision a learning curriculum or a theory coupled

D. Roy (✉)
School of Languages, KIIT Deemed to Be University, Bhubaneswar, India
e-mail: debanjali.roykso1@kiit.ac.in

A. Choudhury et al. (eds.), *Evolution of Digitized Societies Through Advanced Technologies*, Advanced Technologies and Societal Change,
https://doi.org/10.1007/978-981-19-2984-7_5

with modern technology is to "transform how we think about learning and how we practice our profession" [2, p. 2]. To serve its true purpose, new learning theories and curricula involving technology should delimit technology-mediated education from approaching technology as a mere interface in the educational process, a tool to chaperone traditional, teacher-centered, didactic teaching and attempt a paradigmatic shift from learning 'by' media to learning 'in' media. However, regrettably, as noted by most curriculum designers and theorists, the theoretical underpinnings of digital education worldwide have failed to fully utilize the "transformative potential" of technology beyond qualitative change; and thus, there is an urgent need to reassess the pedagogic principles and practices and reconstruct the curriculum in "relation to the opportunities afforded by online technologies" [2, pp. 2–3].

The urgency to re-evaluate the existing curriculum of digital education experienced an unforeseen acceleration by the outbreak of COVID-19 virus worldwide and its impact on almost all known structures defining human existence. Declared a "pandemic" by the World Health Organization on the afternoon of March 11, 2020, this outbreak affected and continues to affect the global economy, health, sociocultural constructs, and education. Clueless about combating the contagion or devising a cure, the world leaders and governments imposed lockdowns and COVID restrictions across the globe. Simultaneously, several people lost their jobs, workplaces shut down, and trade and commerce were highly affected. According to the World Health Organization, almost 200 million people worldwide have been infected by the deadly virus whereas more than 4 million people have already lost their lives [4]. Outbreak of the pandemic has also stirred up massive change and has overhauled the education system including the pedagogy and methodology of teaching. The spread of the pandemic was so sudden, quick, and all-pervasive that there was hardly any time for the educational institutions to plan, prepare and implement an alternative system which could seamlessly cater to the requirements of the education system and all its stakeholders. Barring a few privileged quarters of the world, the sudden and forced shift to online classrooms was a mammoth infrastructural challenge. Consequently, a large number of students were affected and deprived of education. As Pravat Kumar [5] observed,

> According to the UNESCO report, Covid-19 has affected nearly 68% of the total world's student population as per the data taken during 1st week of June 2020. Outbreak of Covid-19 has impacted about 1.2 billion students and youths across the globe by school and university closures. Several other countries have also implemented localized closures impacting millions of additional learners. [5, p. 77]

In India, owing to its disparate, disproportionate socio-economic conditions coupled with an insurmountable digital divide, most of the schools, colleges, and universities struggled to facilitate quality education under the changed circumstances. A report published in *The Indian Express* notes,

> According to the 'Covid-19 Learning Loss in Higher Education' survey by TeamLease, students' estimated loss of learning is between 40 and 60%, university leaders state that the loss has been 30–40%. However, this learning loss is twice the estimated learning loss in G7 countries. More painfully, the survey finds that it may take 3 years to repair this gap. [6]

This article attempts to examine the case of pedagogic reconstruction in the Indian context by probing into the historical background of digital learning in the country and by tracing and analyzing the impact of the pandemic on the curriculum. By drawing information from educators of graduate and postgraduate levels of education in the Indian context, this article attempts to shed light on issues like the pedagogic mutations that the educators had to swiftly be accustomed to, the challenges they encountered, and the way they coped up. The educators selected for this study are engaged in teaching students of English and Social Sciences at the Undergraduate and Postgraduate level of studies in rural, suburban, and urban private/public/Govt.-funded higher education institutions. In the course of the study, it has been observed that the history of digital learning has a considerable influence on the present situation of pedagogic alterations in the wake of the pandemic. Hence, it is worthwhile to scrutinize the history of technological intervention and immersion in order to assess the extent to which the education system of the country has been impacted by the pandemic and the consequent implementation of digital learning.

E-Learning and India: Trip Down the Timeline

Digital learning or technology-enabled education in India epitomizes the subterranean agencies of politics and economics as it traces the journey of the nation through the post-Independence debates to encountering the forces of globalization and economic liberalization in the 1990s. Charting the evolution of education and curriculum in India in the postcolonial context, Pinar observed that education and extension, the curriculum right after Independence in 1947 swiveled around the "construction of a national identity" with textbooks playing a major role to propagate "Nehruvian socialism of the 1950s and 1960s" [7, p. 38]. He also notes how despite globalizing factors of technological advancement and industrialization sketching the contours of curriculum during this period, the "modernization project" failed to delimit the curriculum from its colonial framework and "upper-caste imagination that had little reason to support the cause of mass education" [7, pp. 38–40].

Economic liberalization of the 1990s radically transformed the socio-economic context of the nation by ushering in the global market and connecting "national economy with world economy as an outcome of new economic policy which has been adopted in 1991" [8, p. 122]. Owing to the intersection of the forces of globalization and subsequent growth of digital technology, there was a proliferation of employment opportunities centered on digital literacy and competence which led to the urgency of including technological awareness in higher secondary and tertiary educational curricula. However, despite the dazzling brilliance of the internet and the possibilities of online technology, digital learning in India continued to remain as an aid, a "support system to regular classroom teaching" [9, p. 270]. Using digital tools in classrooms, initially, was limited to teachers using audio-visual aids, pre-recorded samples for demonstration, and using web resources for reference. With the turn of the millennium and the global urgency for blending technology in classroom teaching, the Indian education system called for a scrutiny of the objectives of the pedagogic practices and recognized the need for updating the curriculum to meet global standards. Technology-enabled education was envisaged as the future of learning both by educators who comprehended the contextual significance of a constructivist classroom and academic administrators who foresaw in digital learning the scope for upgrading the national status in the global context. However, despite such recognition, integrating technology in the classrooms of India was challenged (and continues to challenge) by the digital divide in the nation, originating from the economic disparity across the nation.

Inaccessibility of digital services in the rural quarters of the nation has hindered the use of technology in education in those areas and subsequently questioned the effectiveness of a technology-mediated educational curriculum in the national context. The urban sectors of the country attempted to emulate the global usage of digital tools in educational curriculum by introducing 'flipped classrooms' and 'smart classrooms', but learning pedagogies worldwide were grappling to unite the digital domain with the objectives of a curriculum for knowledge creation and learning theories were constantly changing and evolving to 'connect' the human learner with the non-human learning context.

Digitizing Classrooms: Theories and Practice

Although the internet and digital technology were introduced in the classrooms of the Western countries around 1980s, the new media did little to reconstruct traditional pedagogic practices; "computer applications that were used in the classrooms were copies of approaches that teachers had used, and in some cases, had stopped using over the years" [10, p. 2]. With the "socioeconomic shift from the industrial society to the Knowledge Age" facilitated by the "Internet Revolution", there was a need to redefine the major learning theories of the twentieth century—behaviorism, cognitivism, and constructivism that focused on learning as an "individualistic pursuit" with the objectivist epistemology of behaviorism and cognitivism holding knowledge as "fixed and finite", one that is transferred hierarchically from the teacher to the learner [11, pp. 13–14]. Contrasting the objectivist epistemology of behaviorism and cognitivism, constructivism foregrounds the idea that knowledge is created and constructed actively by learners interacting with the world around them and reflecting on the experiences; shifting the emphasis from the act of transference of knowledge to individual perception [12], p. 53, 13, p. 238, 11, p. 12]. However, despite the emphasis on interaction with the learning context, the central idea of this theory is that, as [14] points out:

> …learning occurs inside a person. Even social constructivist views, which hold that learning is a socially enacted process, promotes (sic) the principality of the individual (and her/his physical presence—i.e., brain based) in learning. These theories do not address learning that

> occurs outside of people (i.e. learning that is stored and manipulated by technology). [14, p. 3]

Such a statement underscores the need for new theoretical lenses to observe and analyze the changing society vis-à-vis educational goals and objectives in order to propose reconfiguration of the existing curriculum. Thus, major learning theories like Collaborativism, Sociomaterialism, and Connectivism attempt to address the learning objectives, learners' needs, and pedagogic principles in a learning context that is defined by a digital exchange. Connectivism and Collaborativism (previously known as Online Collaborative Learning) are two significant learning theories that developed from critical analysis and exploration of the digital learning context.

'Connectivism' was proposed as a learning theory for the digital age by George Siemens in a post to his blog on elearnspace.org (2004) and later supported by Stephen Downes in 2005 [11, p. 81]. Siemens defined Connectivism as "the integration of principles explored by chaos, network, and complexity and self-organization theories," elaborating how

> ...learning is a process that occurs within nebulous environments of shifting core elements – not entirely under the control of the individual. Learning (defined as actionable knowledge) can reside outside of ourselves (within an organization or a database), is focused on connecting specialized information sets, and the connections that enable us to learn more are more important than our current state of knowing." [14], p. 5]

Originating as a concept of "self-organised learning", connectivism evolved and emphasized network-based learning, arguing that "learning is a process of connecting with nodes of information and that learning resides not only in the human learner but also in non-human appliances" [11, p. 14]. The learning process is cyclical in nature as learners who have connected to networks and found information, modify their beliefs and connect to a similar or different network to find new information thereby learning via connected points of information [12, p. 65]. Promoting the concept of network-organized online courses as in MOOCs (Massive Open Online Courses), connectivism traced the path to personalized learning environments controlled by "network intelligence" but failed to design and define a consistent pedagogy [11, p. 98].

In the late 1990s and early 2000s, TEL and online learning became synonymous with asynchronous learning domains like Moodle and Blackboard; which were designed along with constructivist learning theories, allowing the learning space to be utilized by the instructor and learners as discussion forums, close forums for class activities and "knowledge building interactions" [11, p. 78]. These digital tools that have been extensively used in classroom pedagogies in the last few years are referred to as Web 2.0 delineating the shift of pedagogic practices from traditional, unilateral lecture-dependent classrooms to an interactive and collaborative context. Some digital tools used frequently in technology-enabled classrooms are video sharing sites (e.g., YouTube), content creation, and blogging platforms like WordPress, Blendspace, and Padlets. These digital tools, at the heart of constructivist online learning, have been extensively employed or envisaged to be employed in classroom pedagogy by facilitators during the COVID context.

Interestingly, despite the promises of potential of these digital tools in the context of learning, a major challenge that instructors are facing or rather, have been facing while implementing Web 2.0 in the classroom was a well-designed curriculum to prevent these tools from being adjunct to conventional modes of teaching. Litchfield et al. [15] observed: "A body of knowledge of learning and teaching principles and strategies is urgently needed to inform teachers wishing to utilize innovative mobile technologies and also to inform the development of national policy and pedagogical approaches about emerging mobile devices" (p. 591).

Pandemic and Pedagogy: The Indian Story

Changing Contexts

Online learning in India in its initial phase was marked by uncertainties and anxieties from the end of both instructors and learners as has been deemed natural by Everett Rogers in his Diffusion theory where he reflects on the anxieties generated "in the minds of potentials adopters" by a "technological innovation" [16, p. 13]. Rogers associates the 'diffusion' of 'innovations' as "a kind of *social change,* defined as the process by which alteration occurs in the structure and function of a social system. When new ideas are invented, diffused, and are adopted or rejected, leading to certain consequences, social change occurs" [16, p. 6]. Such bias and anxiety delineate the interplay of intricately interconnected socio-political and economic factors in the educational context of India. Digital divide, owing to economic disparities between rural and urban sectors of the nation, has remained a major roadblock in the implementation of online learning and curricular upgradation. The lack of technological infrastructure contributed to the instructors' bias against technology-mediated learning processes and lack of awareness regarding updated learning theories and pedagogic practices involved in the integration of digital tools in the educational context.

In the last 5 years, however, there has been a notable enthusiasm in implementing the constructivist models in online learning contexts by educational practitioners in India. Activated by the digital revolution in the nation causing digital networks reaching the lowest rungs of society, infinite possibilities of the internet have been unfurled making it one of the fastest-growing markets for digital consumption. By 2018, there were as many as "560 million internet subscribers" in the country, and academic administrators, curriculum designers, and instructors were promoting digital learning in the secondary, higher secondary, and tertiary levels of education [17, p. 1]. Designed along connectivist pedagogies, the Ministry of Human Resource Development, India and AICTE (All India Council for Technical Education) was sponsoring the creation of MOOCs that would be readily available in an integrated platform named SWAYAM (Study Webs of Active Learning for Young Aspiring

Minds). Offering more than 2000 free courses, SWAYAM aimed to encourage personalized and synchronous learning among learners from secondary to tertiary levels of education as well as in-service educational professionals.

COVID-19 and Constructivist Curriculum

Constructivist learning theories have dominated curriculum design ever since the need for a curricular mutation to suit the needs and goals of present-day learners in India was envisaged. However, the pandemic caused a paradigm shift by radically altering the dimensions, theoretical assumptions and practical implications of curriculum. In a country like India, where education and curriculum are intricately enmeshed in socioeconomic politics, envisaging a constructivist curriculum in digital medium in the context of a global crisis was bound to be fraught with uncertainties, speculations, and, most importantly, experimentations.

In India, with the announcement of a nationwide lockdown from March 25, 2020, (Lockdown 1.0) to combat the COVID crisis, all educational institutions were closed. With schools, colleges, and universities suddenly shutting their campuses to prevent contagion, there was a general sense of panic that percolated down from the highest stakeholders of the educational system to the lowest. With on-campus learning no longer an option, digital learning was deemed to be the only option available. Learning Management Systems (LMS) like Microsoft Teams, Google LMS, Zoom video calls, and Moodle started replacing brick and mortar classrooms overnight. However, this overnight mutation in the mode of teaching was mostly restricted to the city-based and/or private-owned educational institutions owing to intersecting discourses of nationwide economic and digital divide (accentuated in this moment of crisis), nuances of private and public education across the country and most significantly, the *readiness* of the existing curriculum to adapt to changes. Such an observation recalls the central objective of the article—the attempt to explore (a) the perspective of the teachers (in the Indian context) who are adapting/have adapted to a completely online mode of teaching, (b) the effectiveness of the digital medium in designing a curriculum based on connectivist ideas, and (c) challenges of pedagogic mutations in the context of the pandemic.

Literature Review and Hypothesis

In order to have a comprehensive understanding of the impact of the pandemic on curriculum, besides having a prior knowledge of the constructivist principles of curriculum design in the digital domain, it was important to consult contemporary academic reports, notices, and researches conducted in this area, grounded in the Indian context. This article draws ideas and observations from *An analysis of COVID-19 Impacts On Indian Education System* by Mukesh [18], *Impact of COVID-19 on*

Education Sector in India by Prof. Priyanka Pandita Koul, Prof. Omkar Jagdish Bapat, and *Impact of COVID-19 on higher education in India* by Pravat Kumar Jena. Rawal's article attempted to have a holistic idea of the challenges faced by the national education system in the wake of COVID-19 from the perspective of both teachers and students and sought to find out ways how the negative impact of the pandemic on education could be alleviated. Drawn from his own findings, the article does provide a view of the impact of suddenness of this shift from offline to online teaching–learning on both teachers and students but fails to provide information relating to measures being undertaken and/or pedagogical changes attempted by the course facilitators. Prof. Koul and Prof. Bapat's article on the impact of the pandemic on higher education in India is a study based on the challenges of e-learning in the Indian context, one that delineates both the negative impacts of digital learning at the present moment and positive opportunities that this shift to digital domain can bestow on educational context of the nation. An extensive study on pedagogic challenges and opportunities, this study too does not throw much light on either the methods and innovations in such methods that teachers are implementing in an online classroom or do they have records of real-time experiences faced by the teachers. The article by Pravat Kumar Jena touches on some of the most crucial points of observation of the impact of the pandemic on Indian pedagogic structure but his findings too are mostly drawn from reports and articles and does not take into account authentic experiences of either students or teachers. Thus, records of authentic experiences of teachers facilitating online education in the pandemic context were deemed integral to address the three-fold inquiry that comprises the crux of my article. It was hypothesized that the sudden shift from 'normal' classrooms to online mode in the middle of an academic session was less overwhelming for educators who are employed in an urban privately owned higher educational institution where pedagogy was already activity-based and collaborative, supported by the abundant use of digital tools in the classroom than their colleagues in rural quarters of the country.

Methodology

This article seeks to comment on the pedagogic mutations in the context of pandemic in India; how teachers in India were adapting to this new mode of teaching system; the challenges they were facing and the counter-measures they were employing. To have such an understanding, a random sample of teachers employed in higher education institutions (Undergraduate and Postgraduate courses of studies) in the state of West Bengal in India was selected. West Bengal was chosen as the site for conducting the study as during the conduction of the survey during the lockdown, I was in West Bengal and well versed with the pedagogic practices of the state. The sample size was small (21 respondents) and was selected on the basis of the type of institutions they were employed in, the location of the institution, and the economic category of the demographic they catered to. They were interviewed on various aspects of the curriculum they are following at present by virtual meetings conducted over Google

Meet and Zoom video calls and also by recording their opinions and observations by their responses to the questionnaire created by the interviewer by means of Google Forms.

Questions in the form were designed in a way that sought to find information regarding—

(a) The role that the type of institution and/or its location plays in determining the pedagogic practices designed around digital space.
(b) Present pedagogic practices—rationale and impact.
(c) Impact of the pandemic on their pedagogic practices—challenges and opportunities.
(d) The way forward.

Data Collection and Analysis

Out of the 21, 9 respondents were from the city, 9 from the suburbs, and 3 from the rural districts of the state. Although not an equal distribution, the responses facilitated the analysis of the political and economic factors concerning digital availability. Forty-seven percent of the respondents were employed in state-funded public academic institutions and 43% were from private-owned academic institutions (Fig. 5.1).

In response to the question of whether the online teaching–learning started right after the lockdown was announced, 100% of respondents employed in private organizations affirmed that as directed by their administrative authorities, they started taking classes almost immediately after the campuses of educational institutions

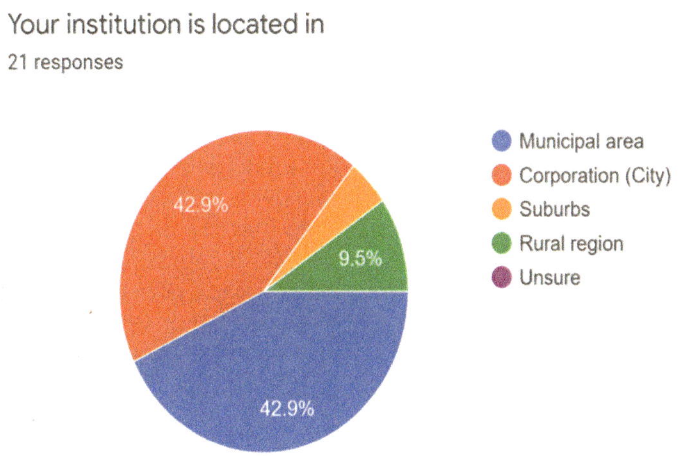

Fig. 5.1 Data collected from Google Form

were closed. Teachers employed in public-funded or Government sponsored institutions, however, noted that they did not engage in taking classes online immediately afterward; they waited for directives from the State or Central administration. The information so gathered from responses to this question was that unlike the privately funded higher educational institutes of West Bengal, the colleges and universities run by the State- or Central-level administration took a while to devise pedagogic methods for the fully virtual classroom. The reason for this delay is, as has been noted by some teachers during their interview, the lack of readiness of the curriculum to be delivered fully in the digital medium. This "lack of readiness" also underlines their own discomforts and unease that characterizes a sudden shift in the 'site' of the classroom. Fifty percent of the total respondents, irrespective of the location or type of the academic institution they are employed in, articulated their unease with this radical shift of learning space from campus to virtual meetings and narrated their initial discomforts in not only designing pedagogic outlines of the courses (that they have been teaching in the classes) for this 'new' medium of education but also employing them for assessment and evaluation of the students. Teachers working in private institutions claimed, almost unanimously, that this metamorphosis of a class into a digitally conceived space did not pose a big challenge to them by virtue of their experience of blending technology in their classrooms from way before the pandemic. This contrastive scenario almost immediately delineates the role of the type of institution and/or its location in determining the exposure to and employment of pedagogic practices designed around digital space by highlighting not only the digital divide that polarizes urban and rural education in West Bengal but also the nexus of political and socio-economic discourses that determine curriculum design and pedagogic practices.

While conducting interviews through video calls and telephone conversations, considerable information was gathered regarding the rationale, challenges, and impact of 'compulsory' digital education in the existing pedagogic practices. Prof. Tanmoy Putatunda, who at the time of the study was employed in the Department of English Language and Literature in a privately owned higher education institute located in the urban quarter of the State clarified that way before the pandemic hit the education sector, teachers in undergraduate as well as postgraduate classes were designing their classes along with constructivist principles. They were using digital tools in the curriculum already; "students usually explore readily available content creating and editing apps to do their assignments," noted Prof. Putatunda. Frequently using YouTube videos and other digital resources in his class in pre-pandemic times, he noted how exposure to such digital tools reduced their anxieties and apprehensions when the classroom pedagogy faced a major reconstruction in the COVID context. This idea was further supported by the observation of Dr. Shrabani Basu, employed in a government-sponsored suburban educational institute at the time of this study, who underlined the role that prior exposure to digital tools and platforms played in pedagogic alterations attempted in the pandemic context. She also narrated the challenges that characterize online classrooms in government-funded educational institutes catering to a suburban or rural demographic by underlining the incompetence of the existing curriculum in public education to effectively blend digital media into pedagogic practices. The reason, in her opinion and agreed upon by most others, is the lack of resources, teacher orientation to digital technology, and a well-designed curriculum that would take into account the geographical and economic diversity of the learners.

The survey as well as the interviews were conducted during a time when students and teachers in the nation were already immersed in the 'structure' of online education by virtue of proliferation of Google Meets, Zoom calls, Google Classrooms, Microsoft Teams, Cisco Webex, and Moodle in pedagogy. This study, using digital technology for data collection and analysis, focuses on the teachers' perspectives of digital metamorphosis of educational platforms in the Indian context during the pandemic. It deliberately limits the sample type to teachers and academic facilitators of higher educational institutes and does not include learners' response as this particular study aims to observe the challenges and innovations in the teaching methodology in online media. Major challenges identified by teachers were how digital education in an economically and digitally divided context affected daily class interactions, brainstorming of discussions, and regular evaluation. This throws considerable light on the conception and implementation of resources and conduction of classes in the digital domain (Fig. 5.2).

Observing the pedagogical challenges of e-learning, Koul and Bapat note:

> In the e-learning environment, in the absence of the learning level, understanding level, memory retention and recall level and other measurable factors relating to delivery and receipt of education, development of courses will be difficult as the course designer needs to be aware about the 'end customer' so that he or she can tailor the course content, exactly as per the students' needs. [19, p. 3922]

However, such an observation foregrounds the idea that a measurable course outcome cannot be expected from a curriculum based on digital learning. This underscores the general belief of the scope of digital learning in the Indian context where, despite attempts to revise and globalize classroom pedagogies, the curriculum fails to update the possibilities of digital media in education beyond its supplementary nature. This was also one of the major challenges identified by Prof. Putatunda in the

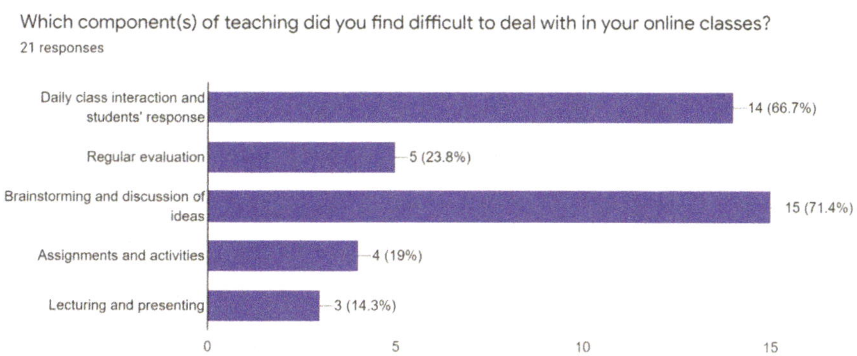

Fig. 5.2 Data collected from Google Form

course of his interview; he noted: "A major gap between curriculum design and technological resources employed in it is the clear identification of the rationale behind employing those particular resources. Educators need to be acquainted with learning models concerning digital education and blend the objectives and desired outcomes of the course with selected digital methodology." However, the need to tailor the course content based on the needs of the learner, as envisaged in the study by Koul and Bapat, lies at the center of any curriculum design and is the most important factor (to be considered) for any pedagogic alterations.

Besides the evaluation of learners' progress, classroom discussions, and interactions in online classrooms (owing to lack of technological, digital, and infrastructural resources), a significant challenge identified by interviewed academic facilitators was learners' response and feedback. Although teachers affiliated to private institutions or teaching in an institution that is located in the urban sections observing otherwise, educators of mostly rural- and suburban-based educational institutes believe that digital medium, by virtue of being an unfamiliar site for education, increases learners' anxieties and apprehensions. They opine that students mostly turned off their videos and did not respond to brainstorming or feedback sessions as they would do in offline classes. This argument underlines sociological concerns about digital education in India, one of the most significant concerns being the unequal distribution of resources. Koul and Bapat present a pen-picture of the Indian educational context vis-à-vis digital technology: "It is to be noted that e-learning access levels are not 'uniformly' distributed throughout the country as majority of the colleges, schools, institutes and universities in the country prefer physical classes instead of digital ones and few institutes have made use of the technology for the benefit of their students" (p. 3921).

The other challenge identified by educators facilitating a reconstructed pedagogy in the pandemic context is the one faced during tailoring the curriculum along with constructivist or collaborationist theories. As opposed to the deductive approach of connectivist theories, collaborationism stems from inductive reasoning, emphasizing the "augmentation of human agency and knowledge, rather than its reduction or replacement by artificial intelligence" and focusing on "approaches and techniques that use the internet to facilitate collaborative learning and knowledge building as a means to reshape formal, non-formal and informal education for the Knowledge Age" [11, p. 108]. Addressing the inadequacies of constructivist theories of learning in a digital environment, collaborationism accounts for knowledge creation by a collaborative network of learners in the form of discussions in an online media where the teacher acts only as a facilitator.

Theorizing the Practice

Pioneering the implementation of online collaborative pedagogy, Dr. Linda Harasim delineated three distinct online learning models namely, Online Collaborative Learning (OCL), Online Distance Education (ODE), and Online Courseware (OC)

[11]. These models of learning with distinct theoretic perspectives and pedagogic approaches have been widely accepted by curriculum designers, instructors, and learners as the future of learning in the digital age. The Ministry of Education, India (formerly Ministry of Human Resource Development), and University Grants Commission, India (UGC), had been advocating online distance education long before the pandemic with its MOOCs in NPTEL (National Programme on Technology Enhanced Learning) platform available for students and teachers alike. Online refresher courses and teacher orientation programs are also conducted to update teachers with the latest technological resources so that they may be implemented in the classrooms. Digital initiatives like SWAYAM (Study Webs of Active-Learning for Young Aspiring Minds), e-GyanKosh, e-Adhyayan, and Shodhganga had also been there to cater to academic developments. However, between availability and implementation of digital resources effectively in classroom pedagogy, falls under the shadow. Writing about such learning practices and theoretical perspectives in the Digital Age, Christopher Jones in *Networked Learning* (2015) notes-

> A society based on digital networks has clearly changed the kinds of labour that are required in the economy and this shift in the demand for labour has an influence on the kinds of learning that are required" (p. 47).

Availability of technological tools concurrent with changing market economy led to "networked learning"; where techno-space became the new site for an exchange of ideas, collaboration, and co-creation of knowledge. Defining Networked Learning as "…learning in which information and communications technology (ICT) is used to promote connections: between one learner and other learners, between learners and tutors; between a learning community and its learning resources," Jones emphasized on the negotiation of technological mediation and human activity in the learning process (5).

This study, along the lines of Jones, argues that digital education in India during the pandemic has been influenced and shaped by certain specific factors. Following are my findings:

(a) There is a dearth in negotiation of technology and human activity in the educational context of India; one which has been accentuated by the global pandemic
(b) Geographical location and type of the academic institution do play a major role in the availability of digital resources which in turn affects the curriculum design and pedagogic practices.
(c) Failed "Education for All"—By failing to provide education to all learners in the digital context due to socio-economic factors, the academic administration across the nation has revealed its failure of conceiving national education along the lines of disparate and diverse learning contexts. As noted by respondents in the study, the pandemic has, in fact, accentuated the digital divide across the state and the nation, thereby delineating unequal distribution of resources across rural, suburban, and urban quarters of the nation (Fig. 5.3).

    With real problems in hand like learners unable to attend online classes due to the inability to buy internet data, learners unable to access digital resources

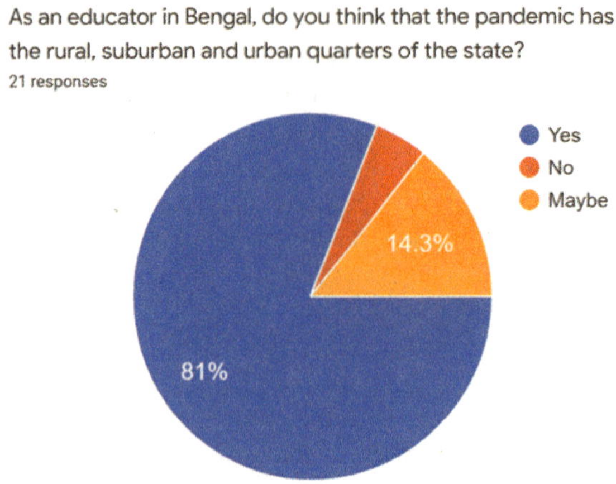

Fig. 5.3 Data collected from Google Form

of education due to the lack of electricity and telecommunication systems, state-level and central academic administration need to intervene and attempt changes in the existing situation.

(d) Although teachers are acquainted with digital educational resources, the curriculum that they follow fails to 'blend' technological potential in the learning content effectively. This highlights the necessity of intervention from central- and state-level administrations to arrange for proper training and orientation of teachers in digital technology—not only in higher education but also at all levels.

(e) The need to develop activity-based learning practices along constructivist and collaborationist ideas is the need of the hour.

The Way Forward

What has been unanimously agreed upon by the teachers who participated in the survey and interview is that even if lockdown is lifted and on-campus learning is reinstated, online learning will continue to play a major role in the educational curriculum. The major reason behind this observation is experience and exposure to the learning context of the digital domain—one that debunks the spatio-temporal limitations of a classroom. During the COVID pandemic, terms associated with digital education as e-learning, online learning, blended learning, Technology-Enhanced Learning (TEL), Computer-Supported Collaborative Learning (CSCL), and MOOCs have become pedagogic jargons of the emerging digital society. Replacing traditional teaching techniques by creating a learner-centered interactive space, online and flipped classrooms have liberated the idea of a classroom from its physical boundaries. Jonathan Bergmann and Aaron Sams, in *Flip Your Classroom: Reaching*

Every Student in Every Class Every Day [20], had simplified the idea of a flipped classroom by noting, "basically the concept of a flipped class is this: that which is traditionally done in class is now done at home, and that which is traditionally done as homework is now completed in class." A significant example of technology-mediated flipped classroom is Google Classroom, a virtual learning space offered by Google for free interaction among learners, uploading audiovisual learning content, submitting assignments, monitoring the progress of the learners, and evaluating them. A site that simulates a classroom space, this digital classroom has been utilized by instructors across the globe during the lockdown to facilitate peer-to-peer interactions, engaging in collaborative and creative activities.

The need for skill-based learning prompted by the theoretical discourse of constructivist principles has catalyzed the proliferation of a plethora of digital tools distinctly designed for diverse contexts. Potential and possibilities of this wide range of digital tools are now being explored by implementation in experimental educational contexts. Besides government-sponsored innovations of learning technologies in the digital domain, private players are also emerging as parallel learning platforms to supplement school education. The contents are simple, can be easily downloaded on a digital device, and aims at the active agency of the learner to 'construct' knowledge for himself/herself. As the learning process is self-paced and autonomous, the learner, who is already familiar with the digital platform by virtue of engagement with the technology in the form of games and social networking, feels more motivated and drawn towards technology-enhanced learning scenarios. With instructors recognizing the multifaceted possibilities of including digital tools in classrooms during the COVID context, the scope for curricular reconstructions has radically increased. To maximize student participation in constructing knowledge, higher education teachers in suburban and urban India are exploring collaborative learning tools in their online lectures. The use of animations (through resources like Powtoon), editing and co-creating video lectures with students by using selected software and technologies are some of the ways how the pandemic has positively affected digital learning in the Indian context.

However, notwithstanding the urban enthusiasm for inclusion of globally acknowledged digital tools in classroom learning, digital learning in India is still stunted by a bias towards traditional learning techniques and skepticism regarding embracing a Western concept. Education in India had been and continues to remain enmeshed in hegemonic discourses that tend to ascribe a seal of authority to the seat of the teacher and construe in the image of a classroom the hallmark of sanctity. Digital technology was long equated with the Western occupation of the cultural and ideological space of the nation, accounting for the slow-paced growth of digital learning in India. However, owing to the globalized market economy and changing socio-cultural fabric of the country, there has been an unprecedented growth in learners and instructors preferring digital learning to traditional modes of learning. As of 2016, "India after US, is dominating the global growth in enrolment" (in Massive Open Online Courses), indicating the readiness of learners to pursue learning in techno-space [21, p. 111].

Drawing from [22], Hartmann and Ditfurth note how, "during the last decade we have moved from a conception of computer literacy to electronic literacy and latterly multi-literacies" that has resulted in "a constant interplay between individual agency and social, economic, historical and political structures that determine the various discourses" [23, p. 19]. This is particularly evident in the educational context of India where debates about the effectiveness of digital learning, as opposed to traditional methods of teaching, are not limited to needs analysis of learners and pedagogic observations but are grounded in political and economic discourses as well; discourses that have been radically highlighted in the studies conducted on the impact of the COVID pandemic on Indian education.

Besides the challenge of creating a constructivist and collaborationist curriculum in a socio-economically and culturally heterogeneous learning context like India, the other concern that involves digital learning is the "rapid pace of technological change" and the way it affects the construction of learning pedagogies [24, p. 31]. Academic administrators, curriculum designers, and course facilitators need to be aware of the changing paradigms of digital education and evaluate their suitability in the learning context of the nation in order to explore them in their classrooms. Despite its devastating consequences, the global pandemic by necessitating the implementation of digital tools in classrooms has not only dismantled the monoliths of orthodox notions concerning digital education but also facilitated a paradigmatic shift in conceiving modern trends and the future of education itself. Speaking about the global future of digital learning, [22] beautifully notes:

> Constructivism and web 2.0, together, can go a long way to preparing students for the digitally driven, post-industrial world into which they'll graduate—a world where our understandings of knowledge, culture, truth and authority are in the process of being rewritten. (p. 28)

References

1. Johnston, B., MacNeill, S., Smyth, K.: Conceptualising the Digital University: The Intersection of Policy, Pedagogy and Practice (Digital Education and Learning). Palgrave Macmillan, USA (2020)
2. Harasim, L.M.: Learning Theory and Online Technologies, 2nd edn. Routledge, USA (2017)
3. Hall, T.: Education, Narrative Technologies and Digital Learning: Designing Storytelling for Creativity with Computing (Digital Education and Learning), 1st edn. Palgrave Macmillan, UK (2018)
4. WHO Coronavirus (COVID-19) Dashboard. With Vaccination Data (2021). https://www.covid19.who.int/
5. Jena, P.K.: Impact of covid-19 on higher education in India. Int. J. Adv. Educ. Res. **5**(3), 77–81 (2020). https://www.files.osf.io/v1/resources/jg8fr/providers/osfstorage/5ef079ab145b1a019e52c0b0?action=download&direct&version=1
6. % university students in India faced learning loss during Covid: Survey. The Indian Express (2021, July 14). https://www.indianexpress.com/article/education/85-per-cent-university-students-in-india-faced-learning-loss-during-covid-survey-7404048/
7. Pinar, W.: Curriculum Studies in India. Palgrave Macmillan, USA (2015)

8. Meenu. Impact of globalisation and liberalisation on Indian administration. Int. J. Market. Fin. Serv. Manage. Res. **2**(9), 120–125 (2013). http://www.indianresearchjournals.com/pdf/IJMFSMR/2013/September/13.pdf
9. UshaBala, A.: Computer Assisted Language Learning (CALL) Materials for Indian Students: A Study (Doctoral Dissertation). Jawaharlal Nehru University (2013). https://www.shodhganga.inflibnet.ac.in/handle/10603/8539
10. Pritchard, A.: Effective Teaching with Internet Technologies: Pedagogy and Practice, 1st edn. SAGE Publications Ltd., USA (2007)
11. Harasim, L.M.: What makes online learning communities successful? The role of collaborative learning in social and intellectual development. In: Vrasidas, C., Glass, G.V. (Eds.) Distance education and Distributed Learning. Information Age Publishers, USA (2002). https://www.researchgate.net/publication/229040545_CONSTRUCTIVISM_IN_THE_DESIGN_OF_ONLINE_LEARNING_TOOLS
12. Jones, C.: Networked Learning: An Educational Paradigm for the Age of Digital Networks (Research in Networked Learning), Softcover reprint of the original 1st ed. 2015 ed. Springer, USA (2016)
13. Hamat, A., Amin, M.: Constructivism in the design of online learning tools. Eur. J. Educ. Stud. **2**(3), 237–246 (2010)
14. Siemens, G.: Connectivism: a learning theory for the digital age. Int. J. Instruct. Technol. Dist. Learn. (2005). http://www.itdl.org/Journal/Jan_05/article01.htm
15. Litchfield et al.: ICT: Providing choices for learners and learning. In: Proceedings ascilite Singapore 2007. Centre for Educational Development, Nanyang Technological University, Singapore, 2–5 December (2007)
16. Rogers, E.M.: Diffusion of Innovations, 5th Edition, 3rd edn. Free Press, India (1983)
17. Kaka, N., Madgavkar, A., Kshirsagar, A., Gupta, R., Manyika, J., Bahl, K., Gupta, S.: Digital India: Technology to transform a connected nation. McKinsey & Company, USA (2020, November 12) https://www.mckinsey.com/business-functions/mckinsey-digital/our-insights/digital-india-technology-to-transform-a-connected-nation
18. Rawal, M.: An analysis of COVID-19 impacts on Indian education system. Educ. Resurg. J. **2**(5), 35–40 (2021). https://www.coed.dypvp.edu.in/educational-resurgence-journal/documents/jan-2021/35-40.pdf
19. Koul, P.P., Bapat, O.J.: Impact of covid-19 on education sector in India. J. Crit. Rev. **7**(11), 3919–3930 (2020). http://www.jcreview.com/fulltext/197-1595749291.pdf?1627773291
20. Bergmann, J., Sams, A.: Flip Your Classroom: Reaching Every Student in Every Class Every Day, 1st edn. International Society for Technology in Education (2012)
21. Chauhan, J.: An overview of MOOC in India. Int. J. Comput. Trends Technol. **49**(2), 111–120 (2017). https://doi.org/10.14445/22312803/ijctt-v49p117
22. Pegrum, M.: From Blogs to Bombs: The Future of Digital Technologies in Education. UWA Publishing, Australia (2009)
23. Muller-Hartmann, A., Schocker-v. Ditfurth, M.: Research on the use of technology in task based language teaching. In: Thomas, M., Reinders, H. (Eds.) Task-Based Language Learning and Teaching with Technology. Continuum International Publishing Group, USA (2010)
24. Schell, G., Janicki, T.J.: Online course pedagogy and the constructivist learning model. J. South. Assoc. Inf. Syst. **1**(1) (2013). https://doi.org/10.3998/jsais.11880084.0001.104

Chapter 6
Problems and Challenges of Social Entrepreneurship from an Entrepreneur's Perception

Kritika Khandelwal, Bhawna Chahar, and Pradeep Singh Chahar

Introduction

Social entrepreneurs address critical concerns of social exclusion with a vision to promote social inclusion [1]. For the new economy, social entrepreneurs are addressed as "social architects" [2], and social entrepreneurship is described as a rare breed and social entrepreneurs as different species [3]. The set of behaviors of social entrepreneurs is exceptional, and there is a massive need to be encouraged and rewarded. Social entrepreneurial activities have been extensively benefited from various confined initiatives all over the world. Scholars advise that people who have the capability and temperament for such work are to be supported to the best by the governments, investors, public, etc. It comes into the picture when businesses assimilate social accountability in their operations. SE is a process that systematically distinguishes a group of society who are deprived of any kind of social exclusion or social injustice. Social entrepreneurs work on the problems thoroughly and develop some business activities set up to help the part of society and control the particular social problem.

Literature proves that for any social entrepreneur, it is not necessary to solve a particular social issue; his venture can solve multiple societal issues for the welfare of people with or without innovative ideas. Any organization that tackles social problems through its business activities, even if it is not a profit-seeking entity, is denoted as a social enterprise [4]. Social enterprises are intended to generate a return for the social order, and if it is also earning good returns for the business, it will be a

K. Khandelwal (✉) · B. Chahar
Department of Business Administration, Manipal University, Jaipur, India
e-mail: kritikakhandelwal.21kk@gmail.com

P. S. Chahar
Department of Physical Education, Banaras Hindu University, Varanasi, India

A. Choudhury et al. (eds.), *Evolution of Digitized Societies Through Advanced Technologies*, Advanced Technologies and Societal Change,
https://doi.org/10.1007/978-981-19-2984-7_6

"win-win" situation for the social cause and business. It is always seen that the top part of the yield of any social venture is always plowed back for the social cause.

Research Objective

This study aims to observe various aspects of social entrepreneurship through literature review. Various definitions and personality traits of social entrepreneurs will be explored with the help of existing studies. After explaining the basic concept of social entrepreneurship, some light will be shed upon three real-life outstanding cases of SE so that the reader can generate a link between literature and reality.

Literature Review

Social Entrepreneur

Many scholars have coined social entrepreneurs from different perspectives [5] calling them transformative forces who address burning issues with their new ideas and persistent vision. Social entrepreneurs are always referred to as people who run business for any social cause which help the masses in need. The practice of social entrepreneurship carries a higher scope due to the significant existence of social exclusion. It ensures social inclusion by solving social problems. The European Commission defined social inclusion as a practice that ensures the gathering of opportunities and means necessary for the well-being of the poor and socially excluded. It is a process that targets such people's economic, social, and cultural lives to enjoy and maintain the usual standard of living. It also ensures their participation in decision-making and exposure to fundamental rights [6].

People who are not hurdled by any restrictions to participate in mainstream activities are called socially included, whereas socially excluded individuals have restricted access to the activities essential to enrich their lives. A group of society or people are usually socially excluded due to different reasons like poverty, lack of skills, discrimination among the society (based on caste, creed, race, religion, etc.), gender biases, physical/mental disability, lack of primary education and other facilities, residing away from the majority of living society (for example, Adivasi or Tribals who live in the forest are deprived of primary living conditions), etc. For the social interest/benefit, an organization is incorporated by the social entrepreneurs where the identified targeted social problems can be addressed and resolved. In his book, R.K.R. Kummitha has mentioned various social entrepreneurial ventures that can occur by different methods.

- **Voluntary Organization or NGO (Non-Government Organization)**: It is generally financed by a government-funded program or formed with the help of charities. In this case, socially excluded or deprived people can be employed in what is referred to as the "Work Integration Social Enterprise" (WISE) approach.

- **An Entrepreneurial Venture**: This type of venture initiates social activities and supports the social mission to support the "donor-based service delivery system" for commencing social activities and creating social value.
- **Creation of Different Social Ventures**: For helping and serving different target groups, different social ventures can be set up, or cross-subsidized approaches can be employed while operating the entity to acquire various finance mechanisms and promote organizational sustainability.
- **Scaled up or Replicated Ventures**: A copy of some good social venture business model can be used to solve the same issues in different geographical contexts, once desired results are observed and initial targets are achieved, for the sustainability of the venture, once again exact replication can be repeated [1].

Adding to the above-shown methods, an entrepreneur can start a social business that uses resources to address any identified social concern scope, necessity, and accessibility [1]. Yunus [7], a social entrepreneur, sets seven important social enterprise characteristics: 1. Instead of making profits, the business aims to solve the problems of society. 2. Financially sustainable. 3. Investors obtain their real investments without adding any type of interest. 4. Profit/Surplus to be utilized for further business improvement. 5. Environment-friendly. 6. According to the market situation, any labor employed is paid fair wages and up to mark working conditions. 7. Work to be done with a feeling of pleasure [7]. Extensive research is into the existence of social entrepreneurship. Numerous authors have weighed social entrepreneurs on various numbers of criteria. Hence, these entrepreneurs are ways ahead than just being an individual or company working not for their gain and just for societal benefits. Dees [3] defined social entrepreneurship as an amalgamation of viewpoints of various authors. He took accountability and discipline, value creation, according to the researchers, change agent and innovation aspect from Schumpeter, pursuits of opportunity from P.F. Drucker, and resourcefulness from Stevenson. The primary operating areas in which social entrepreneurs have tried to bring change are poverty alleviation and employment generation, health care and awareness, academics—education and training, environmental preservation, community regenerations, actions and awareness about drugs, public welfare projects, advocacy, and campaigning awareness about human rights, etc [5]. Dees [3] in his research on social entrepreneurs, he has recognized five individualities of social entrepreneurs, which are as follows:

"Social entrepreneurs play the role of alteration agents in the social sector, by Accepting a task to make and endure social value (not just private value); Knowing and persistently following innovative chances to assist that mission; Engaging in the process of constant invention, variation, and learning, acting confidently without being limited by resources presently in hand, and; Exhibiting heightened accountability to the constituencies served and for the outcomes created" [3] (Table 6.1).

Table 6.1 Definitions and traits of social entrepreneur

Author	Meaning of social entrepreneurs and their traits
Drayton [8]	Creativity, spirit to drive change in society, Strong moral fiber, possession of power, and a drive of not stopping until done are traits of a social entrepreneur. He finds something problematic, not working and visualizes a systematic change to shift society to a new and better way
Mort et al. [9]	Balanced judgment, coherent unity of purpose and action, better social value creation, innovation, proactive, the propensity of risk-taking, and passion are traits highlighted. Social entrepreneurs are determined by their social mission of building better social value than their competitors
Roberts and Woods [10]	Passion, Dogged persistence, Creativity, different vision are few traits of Social Entrepreneurs. Social Entrepreneurship is the 'construction, evaluation, and pursuit of opportunities for transformative social change by visionary, passionately dedicated individuals
Hartigan [11]	Few traits of a Social Entrepreneur are Innovative, Resourceful, and opportunity awareness. He aims at progressive social transformation
Light [12]	Light calls social entrepreneurs Entrepreneurial, Innovative, Transformation, Leader, Storyteller, People manager, Visionary opportunist and Alliance builders. They create innovative ways of tackling some of the most pressing and intractable social problems

Social Entrepreneurship

Researchers, educators, scholars, and policymakers have been debating the definition of entrepreneurship since the early 1700s when the concept was established. The most extensively referred to and cited definition of social entrepreneurship was coined by Greg Dees, Father of SE education, who considered social value creation with the help of innovation as SE [4]. "Social entrepreneurship signals the domineering to drive social change, and it is that potential payoff, with its lasting, transformational benefit to society, that sets the field and its practitioners apart" [13]. Social entrepreneurs are "resourceful, energetic, innovative, and opportunistic" who see the ways to solve the problems that ordinary people cannot [14]. "Often they are iconoclasts" they see ways to do things that ordinary people do not perceive, they desire to do more than building a new business venture or make fortunes [14].

An extensive literature on SE and its contribution to social exclusion is commendable, but a proper understanding of the term "social entrepreneurship" is missing somehow. Many research scholars call it a mere business venture capturing or solving social agenda and some as a not-for-profit NGO—Non-government Organization that works for the welfare of people. Drucker [15] calls "opportunity" an essential element in defining entrepreneurs [16]. In 1987, King and Roberts used innovation and leadership as a core for defining social entrepreneurship [17]. Dees focused on value creation, innovation, and opportunity [3]. Prabhu calls SE a task of social change to develop people [18]. Zietlow [19] refer to SE as a process that adds something new and unique. Ashoka.org (2007) termed SE as innovative ideas to resolve social issues. Boschee and McClung [20] mentioned in their research about using income for solving social problems,on the other hand, Mort et al. [9] have focused on generating superior social values.

Drayton [8] termed it as a change adopted to solve social issues, and Korosec and Berman [21] coined it as a process of ascertaining and addressing vital social concerns, whereas [11] focused on transformation. Morfopoulous et al. [22] define SE as undertaking something accurate, affordable, and profitable to society. The Schwab foundation provided the below definition of social entrepreneurship:

> Social entrepreneurs generate social value through innovation and leveraging financial resources. They transform groups, organizations, or institutions. Social entrepreneurs take risks, act courageously, pursue new ways, and are engaged and committed to creating social value to serve society, particularly the poor and marginalized.
>
> Schwab [23].

In their research paper, Roper and Cheney describe three entrepreneurship models based upon the divergence per the firm's sector; they are 1. Private Social entrepreneurship, 2. Social entrepreneurship in the not-for-profit sector, and 3. Public-sector Social entrepreneurship [24]. SE is a procedure through which people construct Institutions for improved solutions to societal issues, like human rights, poverty, corruption, inadequate infrastructure facilities, poor health, lack of education facilities, ecological damage, etc., aiming for the betterment of life for many [4]. The image of social enterprises has been Blurry and unattractive, it is considered not-for-profit organization, which results in a lack of interest in youth for the same, but some authors have focused on the profitability of social enterprises. In their research Morfopoulos, et al. [22] claimed about social entrepreneurs that they must fulfill the following conditions to be successful: (1) Realism—Business must present prospects that are feasible to undertake with a constructive impact on the society (2) Affordability—Products/Services must be affordable to produce and offer, and the prices must be according to the market rate and consumers ability to pay (3) Profitability—All the products or services should also be a wagon of generating profits (4) Societal impact—The business venture must have a good and progressive societal outcome.

Types of Social Ventures

In 2008, Elkington and Hartigan, in their book called "The power of unreasonable people: How social entrepreneurs create markets that changed the world," have mentioned about three distinct Business models of social-Enterprises:

- **Leveraged Nonprofits**: These types of social entrepreneurial ventures do not have material profit as their goals. In this type of venture, the entrepreneur approaches external promoters for financial help to benefit the public or targeted social group. The best example is Barefoot College.
- **Hybrid Nonprofits**: These types of social enterprises are into existence with a dual purpose. It has a not-for-profit perspective mixed with the for-profit approach.

It generates revenue and earns a share of its expenses by selling off its products or services in the market.
- **Social Businesses**: These social business ventures are structured to realize social agendas; most environmental entrepreneurs adopt this approach to business. These ventures make profits, and rather than returning the profits to the shareholders, it reinvests the profits to advance the social business that results in social benefits [14].

Few characteristics of social enterprises were discussed in a report of 'European Economic and Social Committee': 10 Solution to social problems should be prime objective instead of profit-earning; (2) Mainly follows the nonprofit structure and the profits earned are to be plowed back in the business instead of dispensing legal forms; (4) The aspects of social innovation are powerful, and these enterprises participate in the economy by producing goods and services; (5) Function as independent units; (6) Most often these enterprises hails from civil or related society organizations [25]. There are numerous examples of Social Entrepreneurs and their Social Ventures, which are carrying out good deeds all around the globe, which gives a pragmatic view to the above-given features.

Issues and Challenges Faced by Social Entrepreneurs

India is a land of diversity. According to an article of business, Today of January 2019, 1% owns 73% of the country's wealth. Income disparity in the country is at its peak. India is facing challenges in literacy and even standard of education, affordable Health Care facilities, electricity, infrastructure, sanitation, proper utilization of renewable energy sources, scarcity of food and malnutrition, affordable dwelling, and many more. The problems mentioned above need to be worked upon. What is the purpose of social entrepreneurs? They can become excellent support for the economy. However, there are many issues and difficulties encountered by social entrepreneurs in India. A few of the issues were mentioned by Richy Daniel Oommen in a piece of work that can be briefly mentioned below.

- **Lack of Financial Assistance**: One of the significant challenges that hamper a social enterprise's motives in India.
- **Lack of Entrepreneurial Education**: Very few institutions in the country provide a specially designed curriculum on entrepreneurship. The seeds of entrepreneurial intentions are not sown in students' minds as they are still taught in traditional education practices in most educational institutions that teach a child to get a job after completing the education.
- **Social and Cultural Effect**: Social entrepreneurs face challenges from social and cultural perspectives of social entrepreneurship.
- **Comparative Disadvantages to Business**: The activities of any social venture bear a cost which is to be borne by the entrepreneur from his pocket or have to tolerate some loans from banks or money lenders on high interest rates. Only a

few times, the social entrepreneur works in a rewarding market that can earn him good returns.

- **Lack of Government Support**: The government's schemes and policies are made to support social entrepreneurs, but governments need to work more and more upon a gigantic country like India.
- **Lack of Skilled Manpower**: Social enterprises, for accomplishing their motives, do not get a proficient workforce from varied sources like professionals, laborers, and other community participants.

After literature review, the following other obstacles or challenges faced by entrepreneurs can be found like conveying the business idea to the right investors, attracting donors, working in remote areas, lack of time, raising money, support from established business houses, government approvals, problems in maintaining product quality as per norms, employee sustainability, competition from others, awareness and promotion of business, advanced technologies, support of friends and family. The government plays a vital role in supporting social entrepreneurs; some of the essential aspects are discussed below.

The Role of the Indian Government in Promoting Social Entrepreneurship

In order to excel, social entrepreneurs need a supportive political, economic, social, and institutional environment [26]. India has a magnificent record of social entrepreneurs, and a notable quantity of socially excluded proportion of society in India gives ample opportunities for social entrepreneurship to thrive [1]. The growth of this sector depends on the substantial civic involvement of all who can understand and address social problems. It is felt that the ecosystem of India has become friendlier for social entrepreneurs after independence. The role of government is significant in the success of social entrepreneurs, and the Indian government has initiated many unprecedented steps to nurture social entrepreneurship. Right after attaining independence from the British in 1947, when the first five-year plan was introduced in 1951, the Government of India has visualized the developmental issues, which were allocated proper budgets to the national planning authorities. To promote people's participation in development activities, the state initiated several programs, one of them was creating a social welfare board in the year 1953. "National community development program and national extension service widened the role of NGO". The NGOs were extensively attracted to partner in development activities when the seventh five-year plan was announced. It was a state-run program aiming at "poverty eradication and addressing social problems." By next decade, NGOs appear to be closer to people in need and have promised to fill the gap and be accountable" [27].

The LPG policy that is the Liberalization, Privatization, and Globalization policy of 1991, highly criticized by the pressure groups, has played a substantial part in widening the scope for social ventures by opening the doors for foreign funding. "The government introduced India Inclusive Innovation Fund" (IIIF) to promote social entrepreneurs. IIIF supported all ventures which have profitable and scalable ideas. Social needs related to healthcare, food and nutrition, agriculture, employee development, skill development, energy conservation, financial inclusion, water conservation and sanitation, employment generation, etc., are the main focus of IIIF. Generally, the social enterprises expect the state policy to take up their initiatives to maximize the impact on the masses like the "midday meal scheme." This scheme was initiated by the Tamilnadu state government, which was later scaled up countrywide, but very few know that it was an initiative of a social enterprise called Akshay Patra [28]. The government also helps the social motives of these entrepreneurs by implementing some mandate policies like 'CSR-Corporate Social Responsibility' under the Indian companies act—section 135 enforced in 2013 it is mandatory for any company with a particular net worth to draw at least 2 percent of its last three years of average net profit toward CSR activities.

Exemplary movements like "Startup India" and "Make in India" by the government of India were run to promote and support entrepreneurial activities by offering tax exemptions, providing financial support, and soothing legal constraints. The incubation centers hosted by government academic institutions like IIM Ahmedabad, IIT Madras, etc., have contributed significantly to converting an idea into profitable social ventures. Social entrepreneurs carry different aura. Their inner voice pushes and motivates them to do something innovative to solve people's issues. Their expectations are fulfilled if the real aim of the social good of their ventures is achieved. The purpose and mindset of any entrepreneur is the only uniqueness that makes his company a social enterprise. A social venture has the right to be called a social venture if it solves any social or environmental issue. Profits and money are essentials for sustainability; hence it should not be linked to the purpose. The cases discussed below are of three social entrepreneurs who give the correct meaning to the spirit of the social side of entrepreneurship.

Cases of Famous Social Entrepreneurs

Mohammad Yunus—Gramin Bank

Mohammad Yunus, who hails from Bangladesh, is known as the father of microcredit. He is the founder of Grameen bank. He is a perfect illustration of social entrepreneurship even today. He identifies a problem with impoverished Bangladesh because there lie minimal choices for saving even the tiniest amount of credit. Grameen Bank is an organization that offers micro/small value loans to poor people to support them and build financial self-sufficiency. These people are rejected for loans by the formal banking system; they could only borrow money from local money lenders to accept very high interest rates. Yunus started this system by giving a loan of just \$27 to 42 women of the village Jobra. He found that all the women invested a small amount of capital to generate money like tailoring machines for sewing clothes, earned out of it, and repaid Yunus' loan.

With the help of microfinance, the poor farmers or individuals can take the credit from the bank of tiny amounts of credit as per their requirements at very reasonable rates, which prevents them from going to the local money lenders and financial institutions who charge a high amount of interest from them. This helped the poor buy their bread and butter, send their children to school, and uplift themselves from poverty. Yunus has shared his expertise in microfinance and social capitalism through many books and publications. Yunus brought motivation, resourcefulness, audacity, and resilience to his microfinance business and proved its viability to the world by successfully operating the business for more than three decades now and a vast global network with different businesses ventures who adopted the similar business model of microcredit to their organizations in various other countries of the world. This is the perfect example of making a profit by providing benefits to society. This social idea and his work toward the needy and poor have won Yunus a Nobel Prize in 2006.

Sanjit Roy—Barefoot College

Sanjit Roy, popularly also known as Bunker Roy who was born into an influential family in India and had the finest education opportunities but after college, he did not go to a prestigious career and money; he became one of the most influential social activists of India whose ideas and social reforms are praised and rewarded not only around the country, but all over the world. He is the founder of Barefoot College in Tilonia, Rajasthan (1972). Roy identified the lack of technical and formal education preventing a young generation from becoming doctors and engineers or any occupation; hence this premise was set up to fill this gap of social exclusion. At Barefoot, the deprived, uneducated Indian villagers learn to control "technologies designed to meet everyday needs" without help from "paper-qualified" experts. Roy taught the underprivileged villagers self-dependency and made them take care of their own basic needs, taking into account "drinking water, health, education, and employment." Electricity was used by the college's engineers and architects to power it; now, India is one of the only solar-electrified colleges. Students also installed "hand-driven water pumps" in rural areas for poor people at the unbelievable and once assumed as the impossible height of 14,000 feet of Himalaya. Barefoot College provides night school facilities for children who either perform family duties or work somewhere to earn their livelihood during the daytime.

Barefoot College has educated various professionals like doctors, engineers, teachers, designers, architects, etc. The most important part of each college campus set by Roy is that they are all solar-powered and designed and operated by their former college students. The main aim of Roy with Barefoot college was to improve and develop the standard quality of life of the week, illiterate villagers, and advance the economic production throughout India. Roy helped and supported thousands of people to attain technical skills and spread solar power to the remote villages. Roy won a bundle of national and international honors and awards for his contribution to the society like "The Padma Shree" awards by Giani Zail Singh in 1986, The St Andrews prize in 2003, Social Entrepreneur of the year by Schwab Foundation for

Social Entrepreneurship in the year 2003, The global Solar Community uploaded him with The Robert Hill Award in 2009, etc.

Dr. Kurien Varghese—AMUL

The man of "billion-liter idea," Dr. Kurien Varghese, a social entrepreneur called the father of the white revolution in India, has started the world's most extensive dairy improvement program. Dr. Kurien was the son of a civil surgeon and a highly educated mother. After completing his studies, he went to Anand (Gujarat) as an officer of the Dairy division on a government scholarship. On arriving, he found that distributors of milk and a shrewd businessman were exploiting the farmers. He wanted to help the farmers who were struggling for survival. He left his well-paid government job and joined hands with the "Tribhuvandas Patel" leader, trying to unite the farmers against the exploitation. They started a "Milk Cooperative movement" registered as "Kaira District Cooperative Milk Producers Union Ltd (KDCMPUL)," A cooperative of milk producers or farmers was formed, and now the profit started going directly in the hands of farmers; this was later renamed to now popular "Amul" and accomplished this much-required movement of "Operation Flood."

Dr. Kurien was the man who turned India into a leading producer of milk in the world from a milk-deficient country. Under his leadership, many essential foundations were established, like the "Gujrat Cooperative Milk Marketing Federation Ltd (GCMMF)" and "National Dairy Development Board (NDDB)", shaping the "Dairy Cooperative movement" all across the country. Today the Amul model is replicated and practiced all over the country. This made dairy farming as India's largest self-sufficient industry and a significant source of employment for rural India. It helped farmers with the benefits of "raising incomes and credit and the abolition of debt. This contributed to health, nutrition, education, gender parity, empowerment, etc., as a type of social issue. Many critics do not consider Dr. Kurien as a social entrepreneur as the model adopted by him is cooperative, but his aim and purpose behind the company, which has established the famous AMUL brand with a pious purpose, make him a social entrepreneur.

Conclusion and Implication

All three cases taken in this study are one of their kind, three district examples that can be called an idea of the first of its type. Amul model, Microfinance or Barefoot model, all three tries to strengthen the masses. Amul Worked for small milk producers, barefoot educated rural public, and Grameen Bank empowered the rural poor with small-sized loans. It can be said that social entrepreneurship is about strengthening or empowering the weaker section. This literature review will help develop an understanding of the basics of social entrepreneurship, distinctive traits of a social entrepreneur, and the type of social venture. The definition of social entrepreneur and social entrepreneurship is much more than only working for societal benefits; it pushes the whole economy toward betterment and sustainability, as shown in the literature above.

The reflection of a social entrepreneur is taken as a person who aims to solve some social issues, but while benefiting society, the social entrepreneur can always earn profit for himself, which is proved with the help of the above examples. The surpluses help the enterprise and the entrepreneur to sustain in this competitive market. By providing an innovative solution to a problem can bring in better returns for the entrepreneur. It is advisable for society and the government to support the good motives of these entrepreneurs so that the whole economy can flourish. Good policies and a clear idea of benefits designed exclusively for social entrepreneurs can motivate more and more entrepreneurs to take up the social domain. Further dense literature review can be done on the topic; a broad Indian perspective is taken to explain the concepts based on literature only. Exploratory research taking real-time cases of social entrepreneurs can be performed to know the best pragmatic results.

References

1. Kummitha, R.K.R.: Social Entrepreneurship and Social Inclusion. Palgrave **10**, 978–981 (2017)
2. Jeffs, L.: Social entrepreneurs and social enterprises: do they have a future in New Zealand. In: ICSB World Conference, pp. 18–21 (2006, June)
3. Dees, J.G.: The meaning of social entrepreneurship (1998)
4. Bornstein, D., Davis, S.: Social Entrepreneurship: What Everyone Needs to Know®. Oxford University Press (2010)
5. Bornstein, D.: How to Change the World: Social Entrepreneurs and the Power of New Ideas. Oxford University Press (2007)
6. European Commission. Directorate-General for Employment, & Social Affairs. Unit EMPL/E.: Joint report on social inclusion. Office for Official Publications of the European Communities (2004)
7. Yunus, M.: Building social business: the new kind of capitalism that serves humanity's most pressing needs. PublicAffairs (2010)
8. Drayton, W.: The citizen sector: becoming as entrepreneurial and competitive as business. Calif. Manage. Rev. **44**(3), 120–132 (2002)
9. Sullivan Mort, G., Weerawardena, J., Carnegie, K.: Social entrepreneurship: towards conceptualisation. Int.J. Nonprofit Volunt. Sector Market. **8**(1), 76–88 (2003)
10. Roberts, D., Woods, C.: Changing the world on a shoestring: the concept of social entrepreneurship. Univ. Auckl. Bus. Rev. **7**(1), 45–51 (2005)
11. Hartigan, P.: It's about people, not profits. Bus. Strateg. Rev. **17**(4), 42–45 (2006)
12. Light, P.C.: Social entrepreneurship revisited (2009)
13. Martin, R. L., Osberg, S.: Social entrepreneurship: the case for definition (2007)
14. Elkington, J., Hartigan, P.: The power of unreasonable people: how social entrepreneurs create markets that change the world. Harvard Business Press (2008)
15. Centre canadien de gestion, Drucker, P.F.: The age of social transformation (1995)
16. Drucker, P.: Innovation and entrepreneurship. Routledge (2014)
17. King, P.J., Roberts, N.C.: Policy entrepreneurs: catalysts for policy innovation (1987)
18. Prabhu, G.N.: Social entrepreneurial leadership. Career development international (1999)
19. Zietlow, J.T.: Social entrepreneurship: Managerial, finance and marketing aspects. J.Nonprofit Public Sect. Mark. **10**, 19–43 (2001)
20. Boschee, J., McClurg, J.: Toward a better understanding of social entrepreneurship: Some important distinctions. Retrieved October, 9, 2008 (2003)

21. Korosec, R.L., Berman, E.M.: Municipal support for social entrepreneurship. Public Adm. Rev. **66**(3), 448–462 (2006)
22. Morfopoulos, R., Newman, P., Newman, J., Laube, M., Harper, T.: A collegiate alliance to develop a learning center for social entrepreneurs. In: Proceedings of the ABAS XIV Annual International Conference Limassol (2006)
23. Schwab, K.: Social entrepreneurship. In: Address delivered by Klaus Schwab, Founder and President of the World Economic Forum and the Schwab Foundation for Social Entrepreneurship, at the American International Club, Geneva (2000)
24. Roper, J., Cheney, G.: The meanings of social entrepreneurship today. Corporate Governance: Int. J. Bus. Soc. (2005)
25. Dacin, M.T., Dacin, P.A., Tracey, P.: Social entrepreneurship: A critique and future directions. Organ. Sci. **22**, 1203–1213 (2011)
26. Poon, D.: The emergence and development of social enterprise sectors (2011)
27. Das, K.: Issues in promoting rural infrastructure in India. Gujarat Institute of Development research, Ahmedabad, India (2001)
28. Raina, R.: Policies and the evolution of social entrepreneurship in India: Tight-rope walk to a potential runway. Soc. Innov. Soc. Entrepr. (2016)

Chapter 7
The Usage of Technology by the Senior Citizens: Opportunities and Challenges

Asha Kaushik

Introduction

The latest digital technologies can provide a number of opportunities not only to access entertainment and remote social connections but it can also provide online access to newspaper reading, creating and reading blogs that can be enlightening for exploring many relevant information about the latest advances that are happening throughout the world. This information can also be utilized for the mass update about the latest discoveries in health care systems, trades, market analysis, ordering consumer goods, and online services of various kinds. Digital India, a word introduced by Mr. Narendra Modi, Prime minister of India with a vision to empower the citizens of India with technology so as to simplify their lifestyle and also to increase the employability ratio. In support to that, he launched many schemes out of which online banking, online submission of bills, online money transfer, reservations of trains and flight tickets, and online booking of cooking gas are the primary facilities that are required on the daily basis by the people. This process of online transactions and interactions not only helps in making the life of the citizens much simpler but it also keeps the track record of the different kinds of steps involved in this process and fixes the responsibilities of the involved government officials.

This also helps in creating a transparent and responsible system that is answerable to the consumers and it also becomes a tool to eliminate corruption involved at every step of various kinds of benefit transfers. This arrangement looks quite appealing and attractive but more than 50% of the Indian population keeps itself sustained in the bare minimum livelihood resources. The per capita income in rural areas of India is only about Rs. 24,000/- per annum as mentioned by the World Bank [1]. These people are

A. Kaushik (✉)
School of Liberal Studies, University of Petroleum and Energy Studies, Dehradun, Uttarakhand, India
e-mail: akaushik@ddn.upes.ac.in

A. Choudhury et al. (eds.), *Evolution of Digitized Societies Through Advanced Technologies*, Advanced Technologies and Societal Change,
https://doi.org/10.1007/978-981-19-2984-7_7

given a special status of BPL, i.e., below poverty line citizens [2]. The government has a number of special schemes to provide them support in every aspect of life, e.g., absolutely free medical facilities, right to food, free education, grains, sugar, and fuel oil at extremely subsidized rates. These economically backward citizens have recently been given 10% reservations in higher education and government jobs. All these processes were there for more than 50 years but there was a nexus of corrupted businesspersons and government officials who always used to create hindrance in these processes for their own vested interests. The benefits offered by the government could not reach the actually needy families. Therefore, the government devised these online benefit transfer schemes to ensure that 100% benefits are given to the deserving persons and the evil nexus of the corrupted syndicate is broken. Recognizing that having a smartphone and Internet connection is difficult for many BPL and low-income families, particularly in rural regions, the prime minister launched a scheme that provided free data packs as well as a free handset. Reliance group supported the scheme. The objective was to provide basic Internet facility/connection to almost every family, targeting mainly BPL families and the low-income families of rural areas.

However, many were highly benefited by the scheme but in a broader way, if we look into it we can see that a large ratio of citizens are still digitally illiterate. This ratio comprises mainly people of the age group of 50 and above. A study says that people in the age group of 30 are very adaptable or tech-savvy and keep themselves aware of the nitty gritty of the everyday updating applications they are using. People between the age group of 30–40 are also adaptable at least to the required domains. But people above 50 are found resistant in using the Internet on mobile phones and are still dependent either on the conservative methods or seek help from their relatives or someone especially a youth in their locality whom they could trust sharing their vital information. This information can be misused to any extent and can leave them bankrupt. In either way the outcome of the scheme could not achieve its 100% success. This chapter deals with some of the prospects around the need and the benefits of the digitalization for the senior citizens. This presents the limitations associated with the senior citizens and needs to organize the focused training for them to make them aware about the efficient use of the contemporary digital technologies and the advantages; the limitations and the drawbacks of the use of the digital technologies.

The Need of Digitalization

The connotation of 'Development' has changed over a period. The initial attention of economic growth and economic development has now slowly moved on to include human perspective into the notion of development. Expansion of human capabilities was overlooked when taken in the context of economic growth of communities over a period [3]. Hence, there is a need for rediscovery of the human development approach. The pressing demand for the inclusion of a wide range of indicators to measure the Quality of Life of people is gaining momentum. Quality of life is a broader concept than economic production and living standards. The importance of a better standard of living for people in terms of their quality of life rather than the economic growth of the country is quite important [4]. Thus societal interventions through Science and Technology (S & T) is a significant field of action research that builds on interactions among humans, their technologies, and the environment, and on the use of such knowledge to advance sustainability goals toward equity.

Therefore, S & T based innovation, development, and delivery programs for the vulnerable sections of the society to address problems related to water, food, energy, health, habitat, mobility, and environment services in the context of growing aspirations and quality of Life are to be formulated around sustainability science with new/improved skills and knowledge for livelihood security. It is thus envisaged that establishment of Science Technology and Innovation (STI) Hubs will develop, nurture, and ensure the development, improvement, and delivery of appropriate and relevant S & T approaches for inclusive social and economic development of the less economically privileged population in the country.

Challenges in the Use of Digital Technology

Factors Related to Infrastructure and the Individual Capabilities

The major factors that work as barriers for the use of digital technologies can be categorized on the basis of parameters like motivation and attitude of the user, economic conditions, social conditions, types of information needed, and skills and ability of the individual to use these software and hardware.

Expenditure on the Equipment

Even as the cost of getting information is a crucial attention for many in taking part within the society systems, numerous authors argue that it is a particular barrier for older folks that are more likely to be surviving on their pensions, with tight limits on their expenditure. Despite the fact that there are many developed countries that have developed many facilities (consisting of public libraries) which give free or by charging nominal fee for the Internet, and media for gaining access to the net (along with virtual television), the actual use of these facilities is currently low. However the cost of equipment has a great impact on an older adult's selection to get the facilities of digital platforms has been broadly debated in the literature. Eastman and Iyer endorse that the existing older population can also have more disposable profits saved from many different sectors and could manage the money for purchasing the necessary equipment.

Social and Demographic Elements

Demographic and social factors such as gender, subculture, family standards, educational qualification, and geographic confinement were the factors identified to be related to Internet use. There's little literature about how those factors relate specifically to older peoples' use of the Internet, however, there are indicators. For instance, utilization records display that more adult male users than the females use the net and because of variations in mortality rate difference between both the genders, larger numbers of older ladies usually survive in comparison to men. Older people are much more likely to stay in unmarried individual families and to have lower stages of education than more youthful people. Such factors had been found to be associated with decreased stages of Internet uptake within the preferred population. The desire for being in touch with the latest content and information is evident from the research data despite the fact that people don't consider it as their hobby or they don't find it relevant to their needs. Also, they have specific areas, e.g., unknown Internet settings, privacy issues, possibility of Internet frauds, etc. But a survey conducted by the renowned companies Age Concern and Microsoft observed that one out of four older people likes to spend greater time in front of their personal computers than watching their favorite television programs. The profile of Internet usage for older users is different from that of the younger generation. According to the results of a survey conducted by Mintel about half of those subjects who had crossed over the age of 65 stated that while using the Internet, they do none of the four most popular activities among all adults in the sample group (i.e., online shopping, sending/receiving emails to the family members, going through preferred hobby websites, looking up available official records to update their knowledge). Among older users of the net, in addition to the use of email to be in contact with family and friends, they look for the information directly related to their hobbies, new findings about their health, recent information, and contemporary events. In another study reported by Vuori & Holmlund-Rytkönen found that although older adults strongly felt that the Internet medium is completely designed to cater the requirements of the younger people, about 40% of them felt that their needs have not been taken into consideration.

Learning Potential and Competencies in Older People

While younger people can learn about the efficient Internet usage through formal training or workshops or through the experience at their workplaces, the senior citizens start showing serious issues reflecting the lack of abilities and capacity in learning the new technologies and methods to use the digital technology.

There are several researches exhibiting that many websites have awful designs and older people are discouraged by the complexity of these websites. This reason could restrict older adults' use of the Internet, as they do not like the way these websites operate. However, on the contrary, some studies also show that the older people generally find the use of the computers easy and operate them comfortably. Vuori and Holmlund-Rytkönen found that 90% of older adults believed that the use of the Internet is easy and smooth. While more than 70% of the senior citizens opined that they would find ways to learn the use of the Internet and associate digital technologies quickly and with less effort. In a survey conducted by Age Concern/Microsoft, the analysis of the obtained results showed that four out of five of the subjects (the people who had crossed the age of 50 years) were extremely comfortable in using the computers. It is well established that the older people are more likely to suffer from health related problems and disabilities, which would restrict them from using electronic gadgets and the digital platforms efficiently. These common health problems include vision related problems (affecting 1 in 12 of the population over 60 years, and 1 in 6 of the population who have crossed 75 years). The population above 75 years of the age can also be coupled with other impairments as well. They have high probabilities to have an impact on the ability to use any communication devices, specially the mobile phones as the screen sizes of these devices are small and difficult to operate as the icons present at the screen are very close to each other.

In a recent study, covering one thousand websites providing a wide range of the services, it was observed that about 80% of these websites fail to follow basic accessibility guidelines recommended for the web operations. There are reports that the older population is trying to learn a spectrum of the opportunities available to them through the Internet. Many of them are introduced to these facilities through a course or have been introduced by any friend or a relative. Their grandchildren or children initiated even a few of them to it. These kinds of studies exhibit the importance of keeping oneself updated about the technological advances and the digital world knowledge. These platforms also help them not to become socially isolated either in the workplace or in society. It has also been observed that a number of the older people are intensely motivated toward the use and learning of digital techniques. They overcome the initial hesitation about the use of new technology and enjoy what they see and experience on the screen. They feel a sense of independence and they feel active and confident as they are in touch with their relatives, friends, and family members and in this process, they feel close to the younger generation. Overall, the use of the Internet and the digital platforms increases the tendency to be positive about the things happening around them. The older people who don't use these things and are not confident about these new technologies and do not avail the benefits of the facilities that could have always been available to them if they did not consider themselves too old to adopt the new advances that have become the part of life for most of the population.

Challenges Beyond Control for the Senior Citizens

Health Issues Related with the Growing Age

According to the research data about 40% of the senior citizens have one or the other physical condition that restricts the use of technology by them. This difficulty is generally present and intensifies with the growing age. It may include both types of limitations; physical and mental medical conditions, e.g., arthritis, stroke, Parkinson, gout, severe joint pain or any other type of the chronic diseases, loss of vision, contrast sensitivity, disturbed distance perceptions and even the problem in the understanding the precise speed of the moving objects. These kinds of conditions limit their engagement even in daily chores and using any electronic device that is operated while holding in their hands.

Hesitation in Trying Something New

Most of the senior citizens become very suspicious toward the new advances and changes and hesitate to adopt them. They have many doubts about the new things and are intimidated to use them. Even they have doubts about their own capabilities to learn new things at their age and in many cases, they want to go with their old fashioned but tedious methods as they feel comfortable with these.

Slow Brain Processing and Difficulty in Understanding

It is well known that the older people have a slow brain function due to the decreased formation and the reduced activity of the neurons. Many times they take longer to understand things and sometimes they do not understand it at all. They have an increased tendency to forget things and have difficulty in recalling them, therefore, there may be chances that they feel inferior to the others. If they do not understand the procedures associated with digital technologies, they may also feel frustration. Therefore, a patient one-on-one interaction is required to teach the senior citizen about the use of digital technologies. In addition, the Internet provides a sea of information to the user, which may become useful or confusing, depending upon the efficacy of the user [5].

Requirement of Help to Handle Electronic Devices

As mentioned above that the physical and health conditions may not allow the senior citizens to use the contemporary gadgets efficiently, a help may be required by them to understand the correct use of the mobile phones or the computer machines.

Other Factors Affecting the Digital Literacy

The literature review suggests that there is a lot to be done to develop a clear understanding of the approach and the attitude of the older generations toward digital literacy and the use of digital technologies in their everyday work demands. Currently, the research groups have studied broadly the extent of the Internet use by these senior citizens, specially with a point of view to find what percentage of this population is using the Internet and how much does not. A few researches have also been conducted studies about the use of other Internet-based digital technologies being used for entertainment purposes, e.g., digital television, etc. this is important to mention here that these studies have a common factor, i.e., Internet that takes the central stage even if being the basic necessity only.

These problems except the health issues have a solution in the form of one-on-one training provided to the senior citizens in the form of workshops with the following objectives:

i. To identify the digitally illiterate people.
ii. To make them aware of the digital facilities in specific areas.
iii. To teach them the useful software tools.
iv. To teach them how to create their accounts on relevant websites.
v. To teach them about the importance of maintaining confidentiality of their accounts.
vi. To aware them how to avoid digital frauds.
vii. To aware them about the online tools which may help them to run a business.
viii. To make them a resource person for others.

In the initial stage of the introduction of digital techniques to the older population, an awareness program should be carefully crafted to spread awareness about digital literacy among senior citizens. Awareness should be given on how knowledge of a few mobile applications will make their life simple and easy. In rural areas, the awareness program may also be conducted by the participation of the villagers in the cultural program hosted by the team. Workshops should also be organized for the identified groups making them aware of the importance and use of the various mobile applications. Feedback of the participant will certainly help to understand about the level of target achievement if recorded at the end of every workshop session.

Types of the Digital Facilities Available to the Users

The Digital India dream is about promoting the e-governance platforms that the Indian government has established for a variety of services for the benefit of its inhabitants. These services are especially helpful for the older population as these are available through just a click on the computer or the mobile phones. A large number of the digital platforms provide the services, e.g., ration cards, tenant verification, agriculture related facilities, soil testing, passports, railway ticket bookings, land records, and many more policies. The government is providing about 200 such platforms that are available 24 × 7 and these are really much helpful in making the life of the Indian citizens. A few of these digital platforms are mentioned below.

Digi-Locker

This app has been developed to provide access to the central, state, and regional facilities to every registered user. It connects the user with different consumer support and grievance cells. It provides access to the documents that have been uploaded by the users.

EPFO Related Service

The EPFO app is useful for checking available balance in the user's EPF account. Gratuity and the pension calculations can be carried out on the pension portal.

LPG Services

The registered consumers can book the gas cylinders online and can apply for new cylinders. They can check the availability of gas and orders can also be booked online.

Pradhan Mantri Awas Yojna (PMAY)

This app was launched by the Government of India to provide access to this special housing scheme. This app is useful in providing the details related to PMAY, i.e., application status, subsidy related details, and access to land records via the e-Dhara, which is a special document for the Land Records.

Pan

This is one of the facilities available at the UMANG app using which anybody can apply for a Permanent Account Number (PAN). Users details can also be modified or changed following the specific application forms available at this app. This app is particularly very useful as it saves time and effort for the consumers.

GST App

This app has the features to make the filing of Goods and Services Tax Network easy. The registered users can check their payments just by clicking on their smartphones or the computers.

Bharat Bill Pay Service (BBPS)

Bharat Bill Pay Service is a national bill pay service. This digital facility can be availed to pay the electricity bills, telephone bills, DTH bills, etc. in the comfort of home.

Parivahan Seva Vahan

This particular app is an online service for various kinds of vehicle registration documents' issuance or renewal processes.

e-Pathshala

e-Pathshala app has been developed jointly by the Ministry of Human Resource Development (MHRD), and National Council of Educational Research and Training (NCERT). This is a very useful app for the students. They can access a huge number of e-books, audios, and videos. It has enough resources for teaching community as well like e-books, teaching pedagogy, learning resources, periodicals, curricular details, available resources, etc.

CBSE

This app provides all the information regarding CBSE exams announcement, exam schedule, exam centers, recent notices about exam related processes and general functioning of CBSE, and results announcements.

NPS App

The registered users can avail the services from the basket of NPS app, for example, subscription to the service, updating the scheme parameters, recharge amount, etc. and generating PRAN and password.

Passport Seva App

Ministry of External Affairs launched this app with a motive that all processes related to passport application, its processing and delivery can be used and traced online.

Crop Insurance

The tech-savvy farmers can utilize this app to calculate crop Insurance principle and insurance premiums for their crops. They can bring in a lot of improvement if they plan the crop cycle according to the various schemes that are introduced by the government frequently.

Pharma Sahi Daam App

This app provides the convenience for comparing prices online of the scheduled and non-scheduled drugs before the actual purchase and it is also useful in choosing the substitutes if required.

Conclusions

Almost all the studies have established that digital literacy is a boon for the older population throughout the world. It is particularly useful for those who are alone, live away from their relatives, have mobility constraints but have a zeal for independently managing their life in old age. The exposure to the use of the digital technologies not only brings convenience and comfort in their life but it also provides them a place in the mainstream of society. The older people have a keen desire to keep them connected with the latest advances happening around them and they do not want to be left behind. This is only possible when they have a will to learn and use the digital technologies for this purpose. The world is ruled by the Internet and the information technology nowadays and therefore, this huge chunk of the world population cannot live in the state of non-acceptance of the recent changes coming fast to the society.

If the older adults are encouraged to use digital technology, it supports their mental health, especially promotes self-reliance, lesser feeling of loneliness, and improved mental activity. However, fear of destructive consequences and an insistence for human intervention for the services of various kinds may prevent their successful introduction with these digital technologies. They can also use music and games within online apps or websites if they are well versed with the use of the Internet and the social websites platforms. It might help to revive their mental health and can pave a way to understand the effect of the readiness of the aged adults to engage with digital technology. This population should also be aware of the guidance about the use of the digital technology provided with helpful tools as explained in this chapter.

References

1. United Nations: World population ageing. Department of Economic and Social Affairs, Population Division. New York, United Nations (2015)
2. Office of the Deputy Prime Minister (ODPM): http://www.localegov.gov.uk: The national strategy for local e-Government, HMSO, London (2002)
3. Ng, C.-h: Motivation among older adults in learning computing technologies: a grounded model. Educ. Gerontol. **34**(1), 1–14 (2008)
4. Philip, L., et al.: The digital divide: patterns, policy and scenarios for connecting the 'final few' in rural communities across Great Britain. J. Rural. Stud. (2017). https://doi.org/10.1016/j.jrurstud.2016.12.002
5. Loges, W., Joo, J.: Exploring the digital divide: internet connectedness and age. Commun. Res. **28**(4), 536–562 (2002)

Chapter 8
An Analytical Study of the Roles of Social Media and the Social Development in India

Subir Sinha

Introduction

The development of technological innovations and the Internet system helps to establish a latest form of media called the 'social media'. It is one of the most advanced forms of new media based on interactive Web 2.0 Internet-based applications which tries to connect the entire world with its technological power. The term 'social media' was defined by various scholars in various ways. Shrivastava in his book—*'Social Media in Business and Governance'*—discussed the term social media as *"Social media is described as web 2 phenomenon......Social media includes websites that are available for social networking. They are internet based and therefore globally available unless banned by a government, which is the case in certain countries"* [12]. Miller, Costa, Haynes, McDonald, Nicolescu, Sinanan, Spyer, Venkatraman, and Wang in their book—*'How the World Changed Social Media'*—define social media as *"the colonisation of the space between traditional broadcast and private dyadic communication, providing people with a scale of group size and degree of privacy that we have termed scalable sociality"* [3]. However the term 'social media' defines the relevance and the utilities of its own which signifies as a media for the social purposes.

Social media has now become highly popular and it is used by not only individual public but also government agencies, private organisations and NGOs for various social purposes. However in contrast to social media the concept of social development is wide and complex. The term social development signifies a wide meaning that encompasses a wide range of areas which ultimately tries to explain the qualitative infrastructural change of the society. Social development can also be defined

S. Sinha (✉)
Department of Journalism and Mass Communication, Dum Dum Motijheel College, Kolkata, West Bengal, India
e-mail: subirsinha.2009@gmail.com

A. Choudhury et al. (eds.), *Evolution of Digitized Societies Through Advanced Technologies*, Advanced Technologies and Societal Change,
https://doi.org/10.1007/978-981-19-2984-7_8

as the development of the society or improving the wellbeing of every individual of our society. Social development is a sustainable developmental process and the social media support to bring pace in it. The significance of social media in the social developmental process is enormous as it shows a wide contribution in various social purposes.

Social media is the latest form of media through which social relationships can be easily established and maintained. The prime objectives of social media are to develop social relationships and to promote various social developmental programmes through the use of its wide social network. Social media have the capabilities to exchange information and data from one corner of the world to another within a very short span of time. Social media has moved the world of media a few steps forward. It connects the users to the world and it provides information about the activities that are happening around us. One of its vital characteristics is an interactive feedback facility. Interactivity of social media has given the users an opportunity to speak and to present their views directly in front of the society. It became a platform for the voiceless general public. The views and opinions of the users help to generate the public opinion that makes the bureaucrats and the governments aware of the activities that are happening surrounding us. The interactivity of social media is empowering the public and strengthening the root of democracy.

In the field of social research, social media is a new topic of discussion which relates to diverse fields and provides a wide scope to the social scientist to research and to discuss various aspects relevant to society and social development. The research on social media is mainly based on its forms and elements while on the other it also gives wide scope to measure the effects and the impacts of social media on the society. Social media has shown a significant contribution in the field of social development. Social development through social media puts the light on the impact of social media on society. It is highlighting how various platforms of social media delivering the message and how it is benefiting several communities and the society at large. However, platforms of social media are significant in social development as they are performing their duties in their own style and supporting the development of society.

Social Media and Its Various Platforms

The twenty-first century has shown various platforms or forms of social media which mainly vary in types and characters. Various private and corporate companies across the globe are developing various forms of social media to connect the users just to maintain social relationships and to promote social development. Each one has its own uniqueness, few forms of social media are promoting itself as a instant messaging system while the other focusing on facilities like micro-blogging, video sharing, shopping and marketing, professional job oriented, etc. Amongst the available social networking sites, few popular sites are Facebook, YouTube, WhatsApp, Twitter, LinkedIn, etc. These applications of social media bring revolution in the world of media and information dissemination systems as they are performing various significant functions and supporting the entire globe from various dimensions.

Facebook

Facebook is an American social networking site launched in 2004 by Mark Zuckerberg and his friends Eduardo Saverin, Dustin Moskovitz and Chris Hughes. It is one of the most common and well-known social networking sites that perform across the globe. It becomes the largest social network in the world, with more than one billion users as of 2012, and about half that number was using Facebook every day [6]. The networking site is known for its multipurpose activity where users can post picture, video, written content along with instant message facilities. It also helps the users to connect with various news portals and blogs from across the globe just by clicking the 'Like' button. In the present scenario the role of Facebook in society is multi-dimensional. The social networking site Facebook in over all helps the users to maintain social relationships and promote social development by propagating various information and news.

YouTube

YouTube is an online video sharing social media application developed by Chad Hurley, Steve Chen and Jawed Karim in February 2005. Google bought the site in 2006 and became one of its subsidiaries [8]. In 2020, YouTube has reported that it generated revenue of $19.8 billion and became the most visited website worldwide, with over one billion monthly users [14]. In YouTube, users can create an account and share videos with various other YouTube users. It offers a wide variety of user generated contents and corporate media videos along with various informational videos. Individual public and large production companies also use YouTube to propagate their message and to gain popularity within a very short span of time with a very little cost and effort. It also helps in the propagation of education, knowledge, and various news based data and information. YouTube is also considered as a wide source of entertainment as it amuses its users with various songs, movies, entertaining video, documentary film, etc. The functions of YouTube are multipurpose and its role in our modern society is extraordinary.

WhatsApp

WhatsApp is another well known and commonly used social networking site. It is an American instant message sharing application developed in 2009 by Brian Acton and Jan Koum but acquired by Facebook in February 2014. Initially it was started as alternative options to SMS service [13] but later it shows several functions. It is an excellent form of social media mainly used for communication purposes. It provides several facilities to the users where they can send text message, voice message, voice call, and video call. WhatsApp application runs on mobile devices with the help of Internet service. The service required a mobile cellular telephone number to start the programme and to sign in. It helps the user to easily disseminate any message or information along with photographs and various numerical data within a very short span of time. Along with the information dissemination its role in education, maintaining social relationships and in community development is enormous.

Twitter

Twitter is an American micro-blogging social networking service developed by Jack Dorsey, Noah Glass, Biz Stone and Evan Williams in 2006 [1]. It is a free platform accessible via the website called 'twitter.com' operated through computer or mobile apps. The users can write short messages called 'tweets'. Twitter is available in more than 40 languages worldwide. The platform allows users to consume, create, distribute and discover content. Users can join open conversations as well as watch highlights, clips, and live streaming events [11]. The role of Twitter in social development is no less important as it is one of the vital media through which comments and opinions are shared. Comments and opinions attract the attention of the mass media, bureaucrats and officials along with the governments and help them to understand what the society is thinking.

LinkedIn

LinkedIn is an American business and employment-oriented social networking service developed by Reid Hoffman, Allen Blue, Konstantin Guericke, Eric Ly, and Jean Luc Vaillant in 2002 [5]. LinkedIn is the world's largest professional network with 756 million members in more than 200 countries and territories worldwide. The mission of LinkedIn is simply to connect the world's professionals and to make them more productive and successful [9]. The role of LinkedIn is totally professional which supports the younger generation and the skilled personnel to get their profession.

The Uses of Social Media and the Governments of India

Social media has shown its wide capacity in building social networks which easily engage a large number of the public from various parts of the society. In the age of information, almost everyone is now using various forms of social media. However, the Indian government is not lagging behind in the use of social media. Several government agencies are now continuously engaging social media with the public to share information, create awareness, and educate the society. Every department of the central government as well as the departments of state governments use various platforms of social media to keep in touch with the common public and to provide them authentic valuable information.

Social development is the ultimate purpose behind the use of various platforms of social media by the governments. Almost every department of both the central government as well as state governments has their own Facebook page, Twitter account, and email address which support in the delivery of authentic information, announcement of several programmes and support in the elimination of fake news or hoaxes. Propagation of fake news and fake propaganda is a major drawback for society. Social media used by government agencies deliberately tries to eliminate those fake news and fake propaganda through its random presentation which consist of real authentic information and data. By propagating authentic information through the use of several platforms of social media, governments show their responsibilities towards the society. Government also uses social media platforms to convey various announcements. After the outbreak of the pandemic caused by COVID-19, the departments of the central government of India, state governments, and various national and international organisations like ICMR, World Health Organisation (WHO) use social media platforms for the propagation of various announcements and information related to several awareness campaigns. Social media act as a platform for these organisations from where they convey information for the welfare of the society. The ultimate objective is to maintain social development through the use of social media.

However, the government of India keeps a close eye on social media and on the activities of the miscreants who misuses various platforms of social media for the benefit of their own. The government of India recently developed regulations to curb the misuses of social media. The regulations of the 'Department of Electronics and Information Technology' of the government of India with title 'Framework & Guidelines for Use of Social Media for Government Organisation' are in the form of guidelines of social media use in government agencies [10]. The guideline shows a clear objective of a fair, balanced and unbiased communication system along with the elimination of misuse. The government of India is showing its best effort to use social media in the best way to maintain social development and for the welfare of human beings.

The Roles of Social Media in Social Development

In the age of globalisation, technological innovation brings us a new and modern media system which we call social media. Social media is the media which are interactive Web 2.0 Internet-based applications that enable the user to generate and share content for maintaining social relationships. The communication system of social media is simple and interactive. The information or data posted by the encoder along with the feedback of the decoder mainly helps to generate the public opinion which ultimately supports in the process of social development and strengthens the root of democracy. The content of social media is user generated content, it means that the content is mainly produced by the user. The user may be an individual, a group, a community or maybe a business organisation who deliver the message or content just to maintain a social relationship or to promote social development. Social development through social media occurs with the help of various activities and functions performed by social media such as information sharing, social relationship, debate and discussion, education propagation, community development, online shopping, online professional activities, online health tips, etc.

Information Sharing and Social Media

Social media are playing a significant role in information sharing and dissemination process through its wide social network which Quan Zheng and David Skillicorn in their book—*'Social Networks with Rich Edge Semantic'—mentioned as "Social networks therefore are a kind of lens that we use to discover properties of society, of particular groups, and sometimes particular individuals"* [15]. Information is highly necessary for social development and the social media are acting as a vital tool for information dissemination. Through social media individual user or any news portal can easily disseminate news or information amongst the society. Social media are connecting the entire world through its wide social networks. Information disseminated by social media is mainly related to our modern society. It provides information about the latest activities that are happening around us.

Social networking sites like Facebook help us to connect with various news portals and blogs from across the globe just by clicking the 'Like' button. Public can choose and like the news portal according to their choice. The news portals in reverse are making the users well informed by providing various valuable data and information. However, in the recent days, almost every news papers and news channels creates their web portal and blogs channel to connect with their viewers and readers. The news web portal and blogs send various data and news directly to the Facebook news feed, from which their users generally read and view the news. Twitter is also a well-known popular social networking site that becomes popular within a very short period of time amongst the users. It informed the users about the opinion and views of various eminent personalities and many other individuals general public through a small text message which is popularly known as 'tweets'. YouTube is another important video sharing social site that disseminates various formal and informal information, data and messages across the globe. These applications are serving as a vital source of information which turns the society into an information and knowledge-based society. During the pandemic of COVID-19, social media played a significant role in the communication process. During the pandemic period most of the Indians remained within their home to stay safe from the infection of corona virus and maintained a social distance. Communication system of social media minimises the gap and helps the Indian citizen to communicate with their close and loved ones. In India, it was clearly exposed by several researches that there was a sharp rise in the users of social media during the pandemic period of COVID-19 and in most cases it was used for communication and information dissemination purposes.

Social Relationship and Social Media

Social media which is based on web 2.0 applications that enable the user to generate and share content for maintaining social relationships. In the opening chapter of the book—*'Social Media and personal Relationships: Online Intimacies and Networked Friendship'*—the author marked a significant change in personal life of late modernity as *'One of the most striking changes in personal life during the late modernity is the use of social media for conducting personal relationship'* [2]. Social media helps to develop and promote a harmonic social relationship amongst its users. Through social media one can talk directly through messages or chat. Interactivity plays a vital role in the communication process of social media. The communication process of the social media is interactive, after receiving or decoding the message from the sender, the receiver or decoder can send instant feedback through an interactive communication system. Social media also provides the facilities of video chat where the sender and receiver are involved in a communication process and can see each other while chatting. The system of social media brings the user close to one another. In social media, the public can create or join groups and communities according to their choice and requirement. The group are categorised on education and higher education, health and hygiene, jobs and vacancy, personal relations and friends, tour and travel, foods and restaurants, fashions and garments, professional and career, etc. Individuals enter the group as a member who can share and discuss any issue with the other member of the group. It solves many disputes and problems of the members and motivates them to move in the right path.

Debate, Discussions, and Social Media

Social media proved beneficial for the users in various ways, primarily they helped in developing and maintaining social relationships amongst the users. Along with this there are some other important functions which support in the development of the society and to strengthen the root of democracy. Social media serves as a platform for debate and discussions which is highly necessary for maintaining a democracy. Keith N. Hampton, Inyoung Shin, and Weixu Lu in their article *'Social media and political discussion: when online presence silences offline conversation'* opines as: *'One of the most prevalent views of the Internet is that it has the potential to support democracy by providing new forums for political deliberation (Papacharissi, 2002).*

This view assumes that access to new information and communication technologies will provide opportunities for discussion among those who were previously silent and increase the overall volume of discourse around political issues. This view has become even more pronounced as a result of the increase in the use of social media' [7]. The debate and discussion in social media mainly generate public opinion that resolves various disputes of our societies. It strengthens the healthy activities of our civil society. The social media also gives scope to the users to create individual pages for exposing their activities and creativities, the users can also form groups and communities for sharing information and discussion amongst the members. Several informative webinars and online conferences are also conducted with the help of various social media like Facebook, YouTube, Google Meet, etc. These webinars and online conferences are acting as a platform where knowledge can be imparted and the social condition can be discussed easily with the users and participants. Various research scholars are judging the utility and moral values of social media and presented a question—whether social media is a curse or blessing for a democratic society? The answer of this question is highly critical and complex but it is true that social media is serving the society in its own way and giving the public a platform to speak in front of the society.

Education Propagation and Social Media

Social media is not only used for the dissemination of information or for the maintenance of social relationships, it is also used for the promotion of education. Christine Greenhow, Juli Sonnevend and Colin Agur in the Introduction of their book *'Education and Social Media: Toward a Digital Future'* mentioned as *'Today, the capabilities of social media are influencing learning and teaching in ways previously unseen'* [4]. Students and scholars are highly favouring the social media platform for their education purpose. The users of the social networking site and the web portal can share various text, article, video clips along with photographs and graphical representations for the betterment of education and educationists. During the days of COVID-19 pandemic social media sites like Facebook, YouTube, Google Meet, etc. are used for various webinars, where various research scholars and resource persons impart their knowledge and education for the betterment of the society.

Social networking sites like Facebook, support the students and educationists by delivering various educational information. Facebook is providing the facilities to create groups where various educationists, scholars and students can enter as a member and can post numerous data and information. They can discuss various subjects for cooperation and for the better outcome of the education. Along with these the users of Facebook can select and like various web portals from where they receive various data and information related to formal and informal education. Social media for them is serving as a platform where they can cooperate and share information and knowledge.

YouTube is another video sharing social site that provides various video clips that are related to formal and informal education. It teaches the viewer with proper demonstration and illustration. Like the other interactive video sharing sites YouTube also provides the viewer a scope to select the video according to their necessity and choice; they can pause and rewind the video clip if they get necessary. It is totally user friendly and tries to provide full satisfaction to the user through its videos. During the pandemic of COVID-19 the platform of YouTube was used by several universities, colleges and educational organisations for conducting various valuable webinars and online conferences.

Another social networking site WhatsApp with its huge popularity is also helping in education and information transmission. Students, scholars, and educationists can easily transfer any information, data, video, or photographs related to education to their classmates or any educationist within a very short span of time. Students and educationists can create groups and only Group Admin have the capacity to select group members. WhatsApp attracts most of the students and educationists because of its easy functioning and video calling facilities. During the pandemic of COVID-19 WhatsApp was also used by several teachers and educationists to take virtual classes to a small number of students.

Social networking site Google Meet, which is actually an online meeting site, was widely used during the pandemic by the teachers, students, scholars, and various educationists for various educational purposes. They are widely used for the webinar, online conference, meetings and for taking virtual classes. Maximum schools, colleges, and universities conducted several virtual classes through the use of Google Meet for the benefit of the students.

Community Development and Social Media

Social media is providing a huge support to various community development programmes. Several communities and groups are using various platforms of social media to disseminate their message as it acts as a vital tool for message propagation. Social media for them is acting as a medium through which they are highlighting their problems and social lifestyle. Along with these several municipal corporations and local organisations are also opening and maintaining their accounts and pages in social media. These pages are disseminating numerous valuable messages and information across the globe but with specific aim focused on local people and locality. Other than these various groups are being created on social media based on education, research, medical, legal, etc. to share information amongst the users. They are also acting as a group or community in social media. Social media is acting as a platform for them where they can easily discuss and share any matter or issue which they want to discuss. The message or information of social media is serving in two ways in community development; it highlights the issues or the problems of the community while on the other it disseminates various messages and information of government and local organisations related to community development. In community development, the role of social media is enormous and acting as a voice for the voiceless.

Marketing and Social Media

Social media are also playing a significant role in the development of online marketing systems. In recent days, several business organisations and industries are giving advertisements for their products, goods, and services in various forms of social media. These advertisements are easily pulling the attention of the users and pushing them to check the entire advertisement and also to enter into the company's website as the advertisements are directly connected with the company portal through hyperlink. Social media are serving as a vital platform for marketing for these business organisations.

The use of social media as a platform for online marketing is known as 'Social media marketing'. Social media marketing is the latest form of marketing technique which helps to promote the marketing system of a business organisation. It helps to create a brand and easily attract the consumers to buy the product. It is an excellent system that can easily enter not only in the urban sector but also in rural sectors. Online business organisations like Flipkart and Amazon are successfully using social media as a platform for online marketing. They even display various products on social media sites like Facebook as an advertisement and attract the users to buy the products.

Profession and Social Media

In the professional field, social media is also effective and serving as a vital tool for selection and promotional activities. Through social media various organisations are exposing their activities and curriculums which highlight their transparency in their professional activities. The transparencies in professionalism are helping them to grow reputation and goodwill and supporting the organisation to continue for a long run.

Social media is directly promoting the corporate image and identity for the companies and organisations. The organisations are opening their accounts in various social media like Facebook, LinkedIn, etc. through which they are displaying their products and services along with their indoor activities which help to develop the corporate image and identity. The corporate image and identity are helping the organisations to produce goodwill which provides popularity and stability to the organisations.

However in the business and professional sector social media plays various other significant roles. Several organisations and professional personnel are taking the help of social media like LinkedIn for selection of employees. Through social media they check the profile of various men and women and if they find them suitable they provide offers to join the group or industries. Social media are supporting the business and professional sector from various dimensions just to promote the organisation and its business.

Health Awareness and Social Media

Social media also serves as an important tool for the propagation of health awareness and public service. The vast domains of social media are helping several health organisations to propagate various messages on health awareness, hygiene and various diseases to a large number of receivers. Government Organisations, Municipal Corporation, and Non-Governmental Organisations are mainly using social media along with the mass media for the propagation of information related to health, hygiene and sanitation. Social media has the power to deliver mass appeal and within a very short span of time it can reach the masses. The organisations are using social media as its impacts are much higher than the traditional technique and it can reach easily to the grass root level of our society with a minimum cost. The message structure and the presentation of the social media attract a large number of masses and the message easily penetrates in the mind of the receivers. It creates effective health communication. Several organisations have opened their account and pages on social sites like Facebook, Twitter, etc. Through these pages social media organisations disseminate information related to health and health awareness. The message structure mainly demonstrates the benefit of healthy lifestyle and drawbacks of unhealthy habits.

During the pandemic of COVID-19 the social media played a significant role in giving instruction and awareness creation. They provide several data and information related to COVID-19 which was high during the period of COVID-19. Social media is playing a significant role in the development of the health sector through its proper dissemination of information amongst the masses.

Conclusion

The popularity of social media has increased nowadays across the globe. It is trying to connect the entire society through various social networking sites. Social media are performing various duties within our society and developments are its prime target. The two terms 'Social media' and 'social development' are now closely related to each other. It has become a vital tool for social development. It shows its importance in the development of Information dissemination system, social relationship, propagation of education, health awareness, community development, marketing and professional, and in various other fields also. Through the use of social media these fields get well developed and which ultimately help in the progress of gross social development.

The main objective of social media is to disseminate messages and information through the right path to develop an effective communication system. Social media acts as a tool for the wide dissemination of the valuable message from sender to receiver within a very short span of time. The message structure of social media is simple, brief and to the point which describes all the important facts in a short and simple way with feedback facilities which help to form an effective communication process.

Social media are interactive Web 2.0 Internet-based applications which tries to connect the entire globe through its technological innovative power. Though it also has some negative aspects, it is serving as a new tool for social development. Unlike the other forms of media, social media are advanced in nature which gives the user a platform to actively participate in various social issues. This process is directly enhancing the participatory approach of communication and supporting the development of the society. Social media is definitely a gift of science and technology that tries to support and flourish our society with development.

References

1. Carlson, N.: Insider. The Real History of Twitter (2011). Retrieved from: https://www.businessinsider.com/how-twitter-was-founded-2011-4?IR=T
2. Chambers, D.: Social Media and personal Relationships: Online Intimacies and Networked Friendship. Palgrave Macmillan (2013)
3. Miller, D., Costa, E., Haynes, N., McDonald, T., Nicolescu, R., Sinanan, J., Spyer, J., Venkatraman, S., Wang, X.: How the World Changed Social Media. UCL Press, University College London (2016)
4. Greenhow, C., Sonnevend, J., Agur, C.: Education and Social Media: Toward a Digital Future. The MIT Press, Cambridge, Massachusetts London, England (2016)
5. Gregersen, E.B.: LinkedIn American Company (2021). Retrieved from: https://www.britannica.com/topic/LinkedIn
6. Hall, M.B.: Facebook American Company (2012). Retrieved from: https://www.britannica.com/topic/Facebook
7. Hampton. K.N., Shin, I., Lu, W.: Information, communication and Society. In: Communication, Information Technologies and Media Sociologies, vol. 20, Issue 7, Special Issue. Taylor & Francis Online (2017). Retrieved from: https://www.tandfonline.com/doi/pdf/https://doi.org/10.1080/1369118X.2016.1218526?needAccess=true
8. Hosch, W., Britannica, L.: Youtube Web Site (2009). Retrieved from: https://www.britannica.com/topic/YouTube
9. LinkedIn. About linkedIn. Retrieved from: https://about.linkedin.com/
10. MEITY. Department of Electronics and Information Technology. Framework & Guidelines for Use of Social Media for Government Organisation. Retrieved from: https://www.meity.gov.in/writereaddata/files/Approved%20Social%20Media%20Framework%20and%20Guidelines%20_2_.pdf
11. Mission statement. Twitter Mission and Vision statement analysis. Retrieved from: https://mission-statement.com/twitter/
12. Shrivastava, K.M.: Social Media in Business and Governance. Sterling Publisher Private Limited (2013)

13. WhatsApp. About WhatsApp. Retrieved from: https://www.whatsapp.com/about/
14. Wikipedia. Youtube (2021) Retrieved from: https://en.wikipedia.org/wiki/YouTube
15. Zheng, Q., Skillicorn, D.: Social Networks with Rich Edge Semantic. CRC Press, Taylor & Francis Group (2017)

Chapter 9
The Phygital Dimension: Redefining Rules of Retail Success Through Technological Convergence

Mohit Maurya, Sweta Dixit, Neha Zaidi, and Mridul Dharwal

Introduction

Mankind is expected to witness how technology will redefine the way we live and conduct business. Business integration with technology is inevitable while managers seek growth and efficiency goals. Business and technology need to be in sync with processes and data points while producing actionable business intelligence. Technological integration across business processes will facilitate organizing and sharing of critical information seamlessly. See Fig. 9.1 Not only has omnichannel shopping has become a reality, success here means that the retailers must become capable of delivering fast without fail. Technological convergence would ensure access to real-time information regarding prices, vendors, merchandise and inventory managers, accounting and various other critical dimensions. This is likely to bring efficiency in retail processes while making it more customer-oriented. Gaining competitive edge by improving decision making, increased flexibility, reduced costs, spreading out of risk and unprecedented customer experiences will definitely be affected by infusion of technology in business. The future role of digitalization itself is expected to bring into focus various facets like IT integration, comprehensive usage of big data analytics and for strategic and tactical planning.

Consequently retail businesses are making huge investments in technology to ensure resolution of business processes while augmenting customer service levels. Technology has been touching the lives of retail buyers and also acting as retail process facilitators. A consumer can leverage a digitally connected handheld device with internet access and an ability to change shopping behavior and preferences. Technological advancements thus have been instrumental in creating an exclusive, personalized shopping experience while forecasting customers' preferences and

M. Maurya (✉) · S. Dixit · N. Zaidi · M. Dharwal
School of Business Studies, Sharda University, G.Noida, India
e-mail: drmohitmaurya@gmail.com

A. Choudhury et al. (eds.), *Evolution of Digitized Societies Through Advanced Technologies*, Advanced Technologies and Societal Change,
https://doi.org/10.1007/978-981-19-2984-7_9

Fig. 9.1 Leveraging data integration

a. Unified and homogenized data.
b. Cost efficient data synchronization and integration
c. Convenient data discovery and data modeling
d. Consolidated processes and operations
e. Holistic Customer understanding
f. Enhanced quality of services.

needs and likely changes. Handheld devices have boosted internet adoption in all areas of customer engagement—including evaluating and shopping for products.

To transform a retail organization by being more customer-oriented, marketers need to understand incipient critical factors and focus on critical need to improve in areas where it counts: areas that impact your customers' experience [1]. Customers are more discerning these days, and it will be up to retail organizations to cater to their needs and expectations. Tech savvy end consumers intend to have a seamless unified experience between the digital and physical world. They long for one consumer experience that continuously passes from one world to another.

Herein the evolving customer needs in the context of a transformed market environment needs to be known and understood. This would need a lot of data and its usage by the concerned. With customer interface happening at multiple fronts, marketers need to collect insights from different sources of data making data integration inevitable. While a customer is available on multiple interfaces—both physical and virtual—gathering meaningful insights from social media, purchase history, preferences, survey answers, customer service inquiries will become essential.

Digital Transformation and Business Landscape [2]

An ever-changing customer preferences in a fiercely competitive market place has made it extraordinarily dynamic. To overcome challenges retail businesses need to adapt to quick decision making. No doubt a transformation to adapt will offer diverse opportunities to satisfy customers more effectively. For agile and innovative businesses adaptation of technological integration and digital advances is expected to build a competitive advantage the sooner it is adopted. Quite promisingly, digital transformation offers realizations of expectations and latent needs of marketers and customers. This digital transformation has been facilitated by technological convergence which is facilitated by ready access to consumer big data.

Enablers of Technological Convergence and Retail Disruption

1. **Big Data, Data Integration and Technological Convergence**

Oracle the software company avers that big data is characterized by data of more variety—complex data sets from new data points, generated in huge volumes and with more velocity [2]. Huge amounts of data from social sites like twitter data feeds or facebook, sensor enabled equipment or clicks on a webpage or a mobile app can have terabytes or petabytes of data which can be processed to answer questions. In big data, the data is generated at a swift pace and (possibly) processed in real time requires real-time evaluation and decision. Big data also has the competence to not only analyze structured data but also process unique types of unstructured and semi structured data be it anything text, audio, or video to derive implication and back metadata.

E.g. U.S. e-commerce company ***Groupon*** [3] aggregates and leverages group buying through collective bargaining power. It offers coupons, cashback on purchases and group deals to consumers on activities, travel, goods and services. For this, Groupon had to analyze approximately 1000 GB of data day after day. This dataset is humungous compelling Groupon to employ a huge IT infrastructure to import, integrate, reorganize, and study data in real time. This facilitates partner merchants to benefit from insights making it possible to think the way their customers do in a more effective manner.

Marketers have realized that data will be generated not only on customer interface points but also on social media and across the value chain. Marketers can thus use Hadoop (an open-source framework) and NoSQL to provide more comprehensive responses as there is more information and an entirely changed approach to tackle problems. Big data facilitates to construct predictive models for personalized solutions by classifying key attributes of earlier options and establishing correlation between identified attributes and the acceptance of these offerings. Marketers can thus expect to roll out new products and services, enhance customer experience, improve operational efficiency, anticipate future demands, and improve decision-making and much more. Big data can thus catalyze business innovation by identifying interdependencies among people—customers and human resource, organizations, entities and processes and then understanding these insights consequentially.

Big data can thus lead to discovery of a strong business-driven context. This can thus enable businesses to understand, sorting web logs to decipher e-commerce practices, analyzing opinions from social media usage, customer service interactions, and correlating statistical approaches and their significance for the diverse nature of data. Businesses that leverage these solutions and strategies can then effectively anticipate their skill requirements in advance. This has huge implications on the retail service industry. Leveraging and analyzing big data by linking and integrating unstructured big data with the structured data can be incisively perceptive. Big data analytics aims at including more applicable data points to a business core primary and analytical summaries, leading to enhanced conclusions.

E.g. For Kidiliz Group [3]—a French retailer with brands like Levi's, with global customers across demographic groups essentially needs to gain insights of shifting desires of children, teenagers, and adults. This becomes possible only by availing integrated data sets and big data analytics revealing insights having an impact on real-time sales and inventory decisions.

2. **Technological Convergence and Digital Disruptions in Retail** [4–7]

Convergence is the melding of infrastructures, at the content, service, and application levels. Technological convergence is expected to impact everyday lives through a digital bridge while a radical change is brought in the nature of communication, consumption, work and leisure; offering benefits and opportunities to our businesses and society. Roger Fidler in his 1997 book "Mediamorphosis" emphasized that a multi-level convergentworld has to adapt to the enduring demands of technologies, "changing the way we create, consume, learn and interact with each other".

Technological convergence is the integration of several technologies from divergent functional categories resulting in a new impact on businesses and society. An apt example is a handheld smart device which offers unified advantages of a phone, calculator, computer, camera, watch, music player, activity trackers, geolocation and navigation tool, media player and much more. See Fig. 9.2 Users can thus take advantage of allied convergences viz. technological, media, and network. Technology convergence offers:

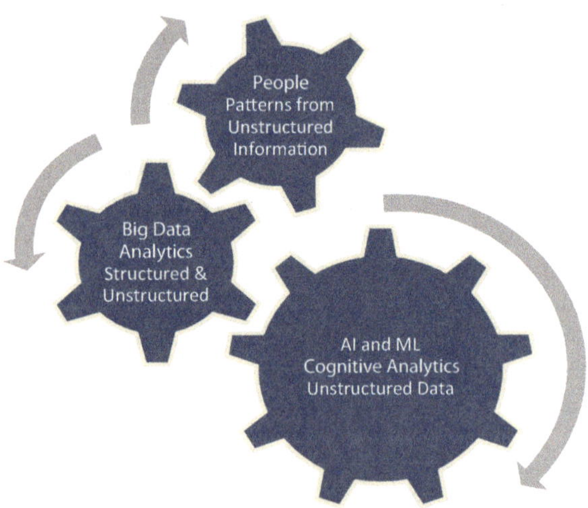

Fig. 9.2 Phygital: An interplay of technologies

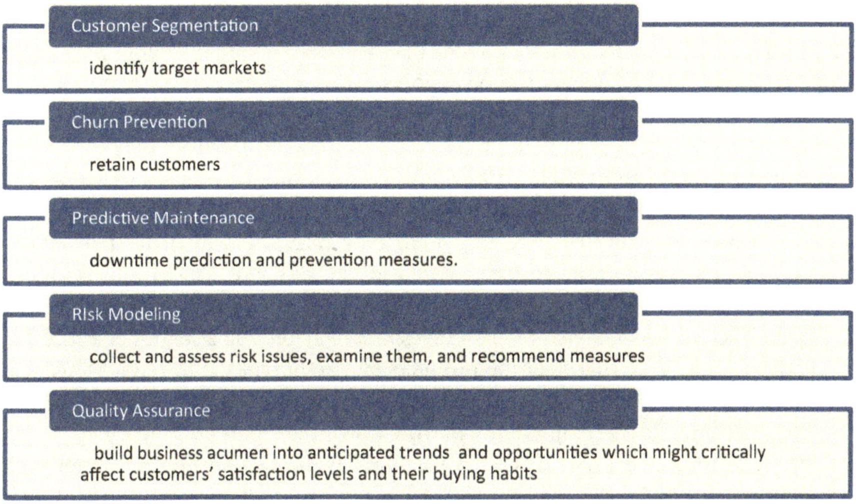

Fig. 9.3 Predictive analytics usage in retail business [8]

i. capability to execute diverse functions to offer a unified purpose.
ii. ability to collect and analyze data of various formats and employ predictive and cognitive analytics. Collected data by machine learning algorithm can facilitate Predictive Analytics tools like TIA or Total Information Awareness [8].

3. **Predictive Analytics and Cognitive Analytics (Machine Learning)** See Fig. 9.3

Machine Learning can be useful (i.e., Predictive Analytics) to forecast strategically vital outcomes in Retailing, E-commerce, and Marketing. Predictive technologies leverage means to anticipate numbers/patterns by means of historical data or records. It can be used for marketing and business efforts to predict supply and demand patterns. **Amazon** the pioneer e-retailing marketer has been availing predictive technologies. Its website displays listings of products/options that buyers are attracted towards and displays a list of products purchased by them with similar interests.

4. **Augmented Reality—AR, Uniting Physical and Digital Shopping** [9, 10]

Augmented Reality does have the potential to transform the way retail consumers buy. Offering an integrated and seamless buying experience across digital and physical channels, and linking them is a test in itself. Optimistically Augmented Reality is a potential solution. AR can facilitate e-commerce by facilitating buyers experience digital content akin to the real world thus reducing risk and doubts before buying. It is also evident that beauty brands now offer the option to try their products on their websites using augmented reality and virtual reality, i.e., *Virtual Try Ons*. Augmented reality has numerous potent applications in the retail sector. **L'Oreal** takes advantage of AR technology by making users observe how its beauty products will look while putting on different options. AR can also endow virtual fitting rooms, for buyers to find out how clothes and stuff will come across without visiting the outlet physically before they buy online. Innovative AR applications on smartphones like Google's ARcore and Apple's ARkit, has given a filip to m-commerce by allowing shoppers to do and simulate the way they do in in-store shopping even before they buy.

Technology adoption by **IKEA Place** gives the option to virtually put and assess suitability of furniture in their home [11]. This is even before physically visiting the store; customers can visualize how their new furniture will fit in their space. This app lets buyers experience their purchase before-hand, try-out and visualize space transformation. Thus AR can conjure up an image of transformed spaces, like the buyers' house, work space or just any space. All products in IKEA Place are 3D and true-to-scale so that later the products can be purchased through their local IKEA website. IKEA Place invariably is a meaningful add-on which builds on the in-store experience by helping buyers narrow down their purchasing consideration set, energy, efforts and time. Buyers can simply walk into any IKEA outlet with a final set of purchasing options considered according to their suitability and their requirement, contrary to a huge number of product options. IKEA Place can help users achieve higher levels of satisfaction with their purchasing experience.

Likewise, ***Sephora, a French*** multinational personal care and beauty products retailer, has a novel mobile app having a *Virtual Artist*. This app uses facial recognition technology to offer users an option to digitally try out options [12]. Clients can glance over the transformation via the Virtual *Artist* app, and can then try on varieties of makeup. If a user seems content with his virtual look, they are facilitated to buy the products. Likewise, with Dulux's app, shoppers can try out different paint colors on their existing walls.

Nike's Berlin flagship store in-store experience is a novel omnichannel digital retail experience. A social media wall gives live updates through social media channels while having a selfie camera [13]. The store has a 'boot room' with a 65″ touch table. Real time product availability (in-store and online) and sizing information is readily available just by putting the shoe on the table, finding, customizing, and ordering their favorite team products. Online purchases through smartphone, and in-store purchases can be completed at the digital kiosk and are transferred automatically to the cash desk.

Brands and retailers can avail AR which is easy, fast, and intuitive while delivering realistic and creative digital experiences: contextual personal recommendations and interactive presentations. In addition, augmented reality brings a spirited side of the digital world. Retailers can take advantage of this tool and give their customers the smoothest possible shopping experience.

5. Impact of IoT and 5G

Significant economic and social value is expected to be realized when 5G communication networks in combination with other connectivity solutions like IoT will be availed. The 5G ecosystem will have various components like (spectrum, infrastructure, devices, services, impact and security) expected to transform retailing in an unprecedented manner. The key functional drivers of 5G will support certain technological applications for certain phygital solutions. Predictive intelligence and operational effectiveness will bridge the desired digital divide. The expected technology disruption of retail indeed is because of easy access to technology and eventual changes in consumer behavior. Retail businesses have thus been investing significantly in another avenue facilitated by internet technology which exceptionally expedites the buying process and is widely called as ***m-Commerce.*** From marketing and social networking apps, proactive retailers across categories are attempting to access customers through their phones. Another radical change which has been witnessed is enabling customers to make e-payments for their online purchases—i.e. shopping and banking concurrently. Consumer and business orientation to transition to cashless banking or e-payments has further facilitated a holistic integration to a shopping experience. *Location-based notifications; live chat, personalized content* and many other technologies are furthering the cause of blending physical and digital marketing together to create a new shopping experience.

6. **The Connected Devices and Omnichannel Shopping Empowerment**

Walker—a research firm speculates that customer experience will eclipse price and product parameters by 2020 as a crucial brand differentiator [14]. Customers will consider buying only when the marketer aligns its message, objectives and design across channels and devices to offer seamlessness and consistency. The internet of things "IoT" is a computing concept that anticipates a world where mundane physical objects will be linked to the Internet with a competence to enrich customer experiences. IoT coupled with big data technology can facilitate capture of micro-aspects of consumer behavior ensuring an altogether new level of engagement. IoT connectivity can create multiple advanced techniques to measure interactions, which means more access to users' data. Retailers can monitor their consumer's behavior, their purchase pattern, their choices, in-store navigation, and the frequency of shopping with the help of IoT connected devices. Every individual customer's activities are observed and recorded closely and retailers can then send them recommendations. Personalized targeting, precise information, good services, prompt delivery and simplified checkout are some of the crucial elements of an extraordinary customer experience, which IoT can facilitate. IoT technology can capture inert, unconscious behaviors and comprehend patterns that can be used as workable information. IoT can thus help marketers understand and find out what the customer wants even before he or she figures it out thus ensuring proactive, predictive and personalized experiences.

For instance, if your smart refrigerator is synchronized with the Amazon pantry app. Your smart fridge can then scan the products in your fridge and find out that you're short on the groceries for the coming week. The fridge will itself add all the required items in your Amazon Pantry app and you will get a message that you have items in your cart please make payment. You confirm items to be sent and make the payment, while the order is delivered the next day.

Converged Lifestyle of Modern Consumers [15]

The structure of how and what people buy, how and where they work, how they interact with others—has been shifting. The adoption of technology has created a noteworthy split between orientation of modern buyers and the traditional brick and mortar retail businesses. The changed customers' expectations are largely based on the technological leap giving primacy to information and convenience while considering shopping experiences. Connected smart devices, wearable gadgets, No doubt, consumers have become used to an array of technologies and devices leading to the expedited evolution of the retail business model. Retail buyers can now toggle from online to offline, or conversely during selection from competing alternatives in the buying process. Potential customers are increasingly adopting handheld devices while relegating personal computers. From online shopping to social networking, users have been using smart devices from banking to entertainment, education, social networking, browsing, collecting information etc. The ramification has been transformation to a more 'digital' business ecosystem amenable to internet-savvy online shoppers.

Another notable mention is the impact of the internet on retailing. Today's customers are likely to purchase specialty, shopping or capital goods with increasing preference of doing it online rather than in a store [15]. Today buyers are shifting away from PCs to handheld devices for keeping themselves updated, accessing any information, for their instant messaging (IM) or any other activities. Cloud or Web-based has already become pervasive even for an end user technology environment in the form of services like email, applications and social networking. Actively engaged individuals on social networks concede to be influenced in their buying decision by 'fan pages' and company websites. Retail consumers have been increasingly using mobile phones to do research, compare prices, make payments, watch live streaming, online shopping, web browsing, etc. Research also confirms that a considerable majority is invariably storing data on the Web, either on any of the options like social media sites, image and video sharing sites and webmail services etc.

Omni Channel Retailing [9]

Consumers' outlook of the shopping experience is changing—and retailers are expected to make an interface available, wherever the customers are. Thus marketers are adopting a hybrid approach to reach out to their customers. A combination of physical retail and e-commerce ecosystem thus, has to widen its horizon and focus delivery of expectations to traditional and tech savvy customers. For retailers, the necessity is to be omnipresent, giving rise to omnichannel retail, in which a unified, seamless and constant flow is ensured to every retail consumer. Here

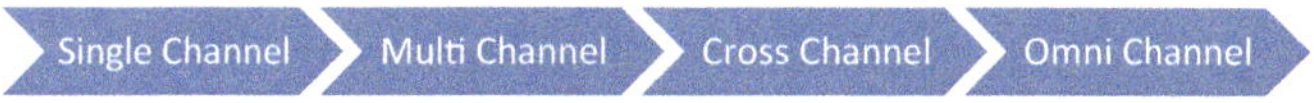

Fig. 9.4 Progression of retail channels

omnichannel refers to leveraging both online (virtual retailing facilitated by intelligent and smart computing devices and social networking channels) and offline traditional distribution channels like physical stores). The aim is to be in tandem with the new technology that omni-channel retailers are leveraging to shape a consistent e-commerce-to-physical purchasing experience for existing and prospective consumers.

With technology becoming more central to our everyday lives and changing behaviors, marketers need to react accordingly. The buyer can opt to buy online from a PC or smart device, or by phone, or visit a bricks and mortar store physically, but an integrated and seamless experience needs to be ensured. In an omnichannel experience marketers thus need to align their aims and purpose, design across each channel and device for a consistent experience.

- Single Channel
- Multi Channel
- Cross Channel—is a strategic, client-focused digital marketing approach to provide a consistent experience while interacting with a marketers' brand across several digital channels. The focus here is on seamless transaction of buyers across multiple channels.
- Omni Channel—The focus is on informational, transactional and experiential retailing leading to improved experience across channels, brand choice and online exchange through the internet or in a physical mode. Informing about your brand, making payments through different modes, ensuring delivery, and opinions about the transaction as an experience should be enhanced. Omnichannel plans define capitalize on the strength of web options along with physical store channels as customers evaluate alternatives while concluding their process of search to purchase from their preferred channel. See Fig. 9.4.

A perfect example of an online and offline mix is **Target Corporation** [9]. When a prospect accesses the Target mobile app and shares his geographical location, he can check real time in-store inventory at the nearest Target store. An order of selected items can be placed via the app to be collected from the store later. This research online and buy offline approach brings forward a new experience which makes the overall purchasing process effective and efficient.

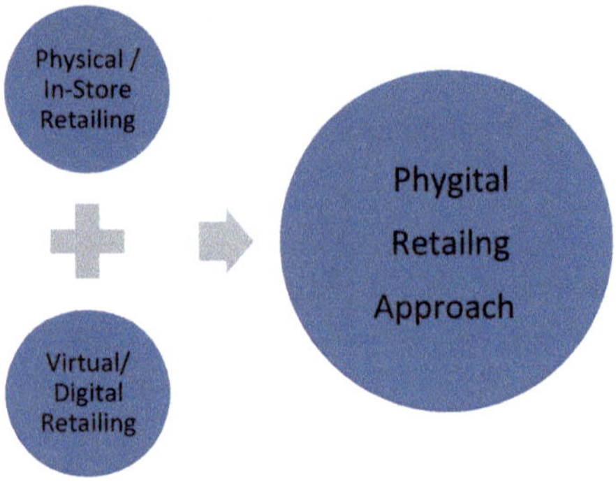

Fig. 9.5 Phygital—A new form of 'omni channel retailing'

Shaping a New Retail Landscape—Concept Phygital See Fig. 9.5

Technology has been relentlessly redefining the in-store and ecommerce experiences with its omnichannel strategy. *"Phygital"* is an emerging phenomenon that equates and equilibrates the innovative technology-driven experience content with the traditional and physical one. It's a fact that physical experiences are more appealing and notable to consumers than the digital ones. But now, digital technology is trying to bridge this gap by offering multifarious opportunities through the onset of 5G Internet. ***Phygital concept*** is the blending of online and offline features of shopping experiences—the physical and the digital. Retail business, as they are dealing with a more connected and tech savvy consumer, is witness to a new format of omnichannel: interconnected or phygital stores. The phygital buyer experience takes advantage of the physical components (the point of purchase, its merchandise, etc.) and digital components (touch screens, web/inter connected mirrors, NFC cards, etc.) simultaneously effectively ensuring a hybrid format of efficient and effective retailing.

From interactive window displays capable of initiating shopping exchange to interactive fitting rooms to personalized recommendations, click and collect, facial recognition, automated check-in and out, electronic shelf-labels, self check out tills, gig style employment, digital signage, global retail businesses are gearing up by integrating cutting-edge technology to create engaging digital experience by availing a hybrid approach.

Phygital Ecosystem: The Retail Experience of the Future

Technological convergence has brought an unprecedented disruption in the retail landscape which will inevitably bring a role change of traditional retailers as a single point for shopping. See Fig. 9.6. Though on-line has evolved as a separate option for

Fig. 9.6 Hybridization enablers of phygital dimension

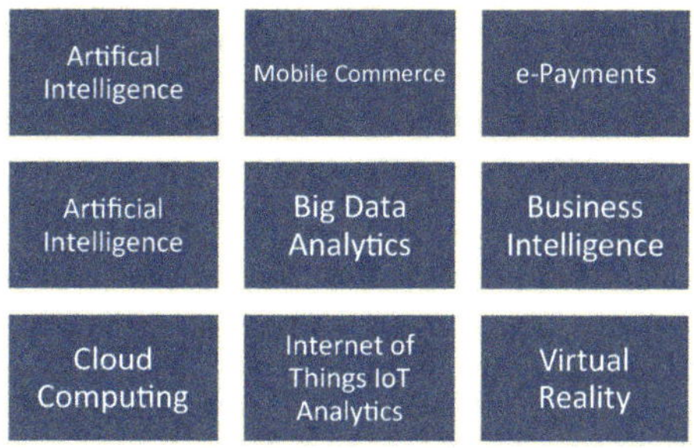

retailing but in an attempt to merge and meld customer experience in a unified manner an omni-channel approach has emerged. The 'Phygital dimension' of retailing has thus been no short than a revolution offering a versatile click-and collect interface to its prospects. No doubt technology benefits can enrich overall retail shopping experience but for this a new operating model is to be envisaged. Retailers thus need to work on process optimisation with automation to enable and overcome digital challenges in the near future. Thus we can expect to witness retailers to adapt to the technological revolution seeking growth, survival and offer superior consumer value proposition.

References

1. Villamor, F.: 6 reasons why data integration matters in retail. Ducen IT. https://blog.ducenit.com/why-data-integration-retail (September 1, 2020). Accessed May 5, 2021
2. What is big data? Oracle. https://www.oracle.com/in/big-data/what-is-big-data/ (2021). Accessed May 15, 2021
3. Big data in retail: common benefits and 7 real-life examples. https://www.talend.com/resources/big-data-retail/ (2021). Accessed May 15, 2021
4. Park, S.E.: Technological convergence: regulatory, digital privacy, and data security issues. Congressional Research Service. https://fas.org/sgp/crs/misc/R45746.pdf (May 30, 2019). Accessed May 15, 2021
5. Oka, T., Ghai, S., Venkatesan, P., Bagri, A.: Disruptions in retail through digital transformation reimagining the store of the future. Deloitte ICC. https://www2.deloitte.com/content/dam/Deloitte/in/Documents/CIP/in-cip-disruptions-in-retail-noexp.pdf (Nov 2017). Accessed May 15, 2021
6. Biondi, J.-E., et al.: Perspectives 2021 retail industry outlook, the new rules of retail. Deloitte. https://www2.deloitte.com/us/en/pages/consumer-business/articles/retail-distribution-industry-outlook.html (2021). Accessed April 12, 2021
7. Ramanathan, A., et al.: Digital disruption in retail. Deloitte RAI. https://www2.deloitte.com/content/dam/Deloitte/in/Documents/consumer-business/in-consumer-Digital%20Disruption%20in%20Retail_Retail%20Leadership%20Summit%202020%20Report.pdf (Feb 2020). Accessed April 12, 2021
8. Kovalenko, O.: 5 most valuable applications of machine learning in retail. SPD Group. https://spd.group/machine-learning/predictive-analytics-and-machine-learning-in-retail/ (June 23, 2020). Accessed April 10, 2021

9. Heslop, B.: Omnichannel retail: 6 technologies to transform your strategy. Content Stack. https://www.contentstack.com/blog/all-about-headless/6-technologies-to-transform-your-omnichannel-retail-strategy/ (Nov 06, 2019). Accessed June 10, 2021
10. Codewave: Omnichannel retail strategy – tech-led customer experience elevation. https://insights.codewave.com/omnichannel-retail-strategy/ (December 11, 2020). Accessed June 10, 2021
11. SPACE10: IKEA place: bridging the imagination gap with AR. https://space10.com/project/ikea-place/ (2021). Accessed June 10, 2021
12. McKinnon, T.: 10 of the best augmented reality (AR) shopping apps to try today. Indigo Digital.https://www.indigo9digital.com/blog/how-six-leading-retailers-use-augmented-reality-apps-to-disrupt-the-shopping-experience (May 8, 2020). Accessed June 10, 2021
13. Marlow, T.: How sportswear brands are developing an omnichannel strategy. Lengow Blog. https://blog.lengow.com/how-sportswear-brands-are-developing-an-omnichannel-strategy/ (Dec 07, 2016). Accessed June 12, 2021
14. Karia, K.: The IoT brings new meaning to the omnichannel customer experience. CMS Wire. https://www.cmswire.com/customer-experience/the-iot-brings-new-meaning-to-the-omnichannel-customer-experience/ (Jan 16, 2019). Accessed June 12, 2021
15. Wright, N., Jin, E., et al.: The converged lifestyle consumers and convergence 5, kpmg.com/convergence. KPMG China. https://assets.kpmg/content/dam/kpmg/pdf/2012/01/Converged-lifestyle-O-201112.pdf (2012). Accessed June 12, 2021

Chapter 10
Smart Is New Green: A Sustainability Revolution with Internet of Things and Fog

Shelly Garg

Introduction

Global coverage has been done wonderfully by the Internet of Things popularly known as IoT where it contains various sensing devices such as sensors, actuators for data gathering process, and through gateways, the data gathered is further processed and analyzed for resolving the user queries. IoT itself says that we are connecting things via the internet which makes them intelligent and by intelligent here we mean that data gathered will be processed intelligently keeping in mind the user's needs [1–4]. To make any environment smart we need the current technology i.e., IoT which is linked with servers, various end devices, infrastructure, and users in a smart manner where it uses the interconnected networks over the IP network making all of them connected completely. This kind of smart environment brings in a new experience itself where anything can be made well connected and smart to fulfill the user's needs.

Internet of Things

IoT is basically a group of sensors, gateways, software, and other technology which has to fulfill the purpose of exchange of data and connecting various devices or systems. Technology plays a pivotal role in maintaining user life efficiently and provides comfortability. Many IoT-based applications have proven to be very useful for users in day-to-day life such as smart home-based applications, online shopping, and smart lighting systems, to prevent human loss deployment of drones in military applications, smartphones, and smart speakers for entertainment purposes. This is

S. Garg (✉)
University of Petroleum and Energy Studies, Dehradun, India
e-mail: shelly.gupta119@gmail.com

A. Choudhury et al. (eds.), *Evolution of Digitized Societies Through Advanced Technologies*, Advanced Technologies and Societal Change,
https://doi.org/10.1007/978-981-19-2984-7_10

a wide ocean of applications which are discussed thoroughly in Section 10.2. IoT's major characteristics and trends consist of intelligence and its architecture which consists of devices, edge gateways, and cloud. Due to a great amount of increase in different links, interactions between various sensors and actuators and its capacity to include more sometimes lead IoT to very complex systems. If we talk about its size then it normally consists of 50 to 100 trillion objects. Enabling technologies for IoT is addressability, short-range wireless connections such as Li-Fi, NFC, RFID, Wi-Fi, Zigbee, z-wave, medium-range wireless such as LTE, 5G, and long-range wireless such as LPWAN, VSAT (very small aperture terminal) and wired such as Ethernet, Power-Line communication (PLC) [5–7]. Due to its popularity, many companies have deployed IoT for their business because of which the government has applied some regulations such as data security measures need to be ensured, data consent need to be taken, and data minimization needs to be done. Major limitations in the adoption of IoT on which researchers are working tirelessly and has also become an attractive area of research which is privacy and security concerns, business planning, traditional government structures, and project management.

Fog Computing

Whenever we sense the data and data is gathered which contain user queries from the IoT devices such as actuators, sensors, etc., those queries from the user end need to be resolved and requests are made to cloud due to the increase in overhead on cloud, a new term has been introduced which is fog computing which handles the user queries in between and try to resolve it out, if possible, to decrease the overhead of cloud. If data requested is not present within the fog layer, then a request is made by fog to cloud for the solution to the query which is then forwarded to the user in the end [8]. As one person today uses many devices which have resulted into generation of huge amount of data as well as generation of n number of queries and resolving all those queries on the cloud has made it impossible to handle such amount of request and hence slow down the efficiency, the solution to this problem is fog computing which helps in efficient resource management as well handling of request done prior hand for time and cost-effectiveness. Many fog and cloud applications are addressed in Fig. 10.1.

Green Environmental Technology

The major concerns are conservation of environment and improving health such as working on the practices such as investment in renewable energy, conservation practices, and informed consumption. Plenty of renewable energy is there such as biomass energy, wind energy, etc. When we talk about green environment technology, it basically refers to the preservation of the environment by reusing, reducing, and recycling

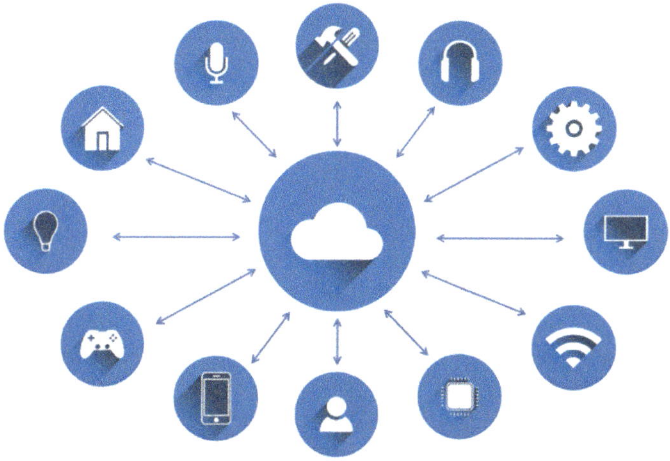

Fig. 10.1 Fog–cloud computing applications [9]

processes. Development of such technologies which can help in reduction of pollution, reduction of waste generation and consumption of resources, and conservation of natural resources such as forests. Technology has played a pivotal role in maintaining a green environment such as the production of organic foods where a lot of researchers have contributed successfully with multiple benefits [9]. Producing many smart applications which can be used only when a user needs otherwise due to its remote operability feature makes it efficient in resource management and energy conservation. Reduction in the usage of paper by digitalizing the complete process saving many trees. Going green can provide:

- Economic benefits.
- Health benefits.
- Environmental benefits.

In this chapter, we have thoroughly discussed all the benefits which are provided by green technology with the usage of Internet-based applications and for the data analysis process how fog computing can play a pivotal role [10–13]. The organization of chapters is as follows:

- Section 10.1 discusses about the introduction to IoT and fog computing, also about the sustainable environment and its contribution.
- Section 10.2 discusses the vast application area of IoT-enabled Smart Environment stating smart is new green.
- Section 10.3 discusses the energy consumption concerns within fog as well as IoT environment.
- Section 10.4 discusses how IoT and fog with other technologies are working hand-in-hand towards sustainable environment.

- Section 10.5 in this section, a conclusion has been done for the chapter with future research opportunities.

IoT-Enabled Smart Environment Applications

Technology has eased everyone's life to a great extent and the IoT has proven to be quite an area where the spectrum of its application is on an increasing graph from a global perspective. Many applications are based on the prevention of human loss, ease day-to-day life, and reduction in thefts, hence increasing the security and automation of many works so that human efforts can be provided in other areas where machines are still not helpful [14–17]. We can see machines help in automation of many areas, but human intervention is still required. Here, we discuss many smart applications which are observed, and efforts are put to cover the maximum of the applications, but still, the area is so vast that making it a tough task for authors but still few of the applications are included in one another and discussed thoroughly by the author [18].

Smart Homes

Presently, smart home applications have come out to be one of the most practical and the best applications in the field of IoT, where a keen interest has been shown in the field of security of homes, convenience which includes smart light system, smart entertainment section where one can record the shows for the remote purpose. One of the interesting applications which has been observed is an intelligent utility system, which contains the electricity meter with an IoT device where it can give an alert for usage of water on a daily basis and that data can be recorded in an application in smartphones for future access as well which can help in conservation of water to a great level [19]. We have even seen set-top boxes in the entertainment field where one can record the shows and the shows can be enjoyed without any location restrictions. Security of homes is one of the major concerns for every user and IoT has proven a lot in that field where we can have advanced locking system which is enabled by user authentication which can be human eye retina or the thumbprint or face scan, if approved only make the user enter any of the building or home which can prevent unnecessary human interventions and various thefts. To provide ease in day-to-day life of a user, IoT has proven to be very efficient as with one voice control lights can be switched off or on as per usage. Not only that, any of the smart applications in the home such as fridges, microwaves, and gates with sensors can be controlled with one voice command. In fact, if one is not at home, even then all these applications can be controlled by a Smart Home App which can be installed by the user on the phone and gives the freedom to operate remotely. It has been observed that connected surveillance systems are also a very effective application and part of Smart Home

System which can provide an enhanced feature of home security. As IoT is evolving and technology is improving day by day, we can expect many changes in future where one can see the enhancement in security of home applications [20–24].

Smart City

Nowadays, every government authority, be it in developing or developed countries, wants to make their cities a smart city where not only the internet access is being provided to the people but to the devices which are there in the smart city project are also enabled smart. Many projects have been completed by various government organizations where cities are made smart where devices are connected with people and users can communicate within themselves in a smart manner [25]. A few areas where IoT-based devices have worked well are electricity management, management of water usage in homes, government organization, management of waste by installing smart bin systems in cities, and management of traffic. It is also one of the aims which can save a lot of time of user and can provide conservation of energy such as petrol, diesel, etc. All these applications work towards providing ease on a daily basis and try to eliminate the challenges faced by users as well [26].

Smart Transportation: Smart Parking, and Self-Driven Cars

It is known to be one of the revolutionizing areas in smart cities, aiming towards mobility, and responding in the emergency situations further with reduction in the congestion on roads. The key solution to this problem consists of sensors, communication with advanced technologies, high-speed networks, and automation concepts which can be achieved by enabling IoT [27]. Civilization has come a long way. Earlier, we used to move via horses, carriages, and camels from one place to another. Now, they have been replaced with automatic, electric vehicles, and with the IoT revolution, the next step to this is smart transportation. As per the US government, ITS (Intelligent transport system) uses various technologies with an aim to monitor, manage, and evaluate the transportation systems for enhancement of efficiency and purpose of safety. In simpler words, it can be stated that making transportation smart is increasing the convenience in movement, making it more effective in terms of cost for city as well as the individual level, and enhancing the safety [28].

Smart Building Climate Control

Ventilation, heating, and air conditioning (HVAC) systems play a major role in the energy usage in the buildings. To improve the cost efficiency of any business this point plays a major role in that. Making any building smart includes the comfort of temperature management but extended comfort includes providing a drier and warm air with the help of dehumidification for summers or improving the overall quality of any room [29]. Also, researchers are working on developing smart windows which can detect the outside temperature and maintain the indoor environmental condition. This window-based application can be of a car, train, any bus, or public and private transport which can help to a great extent in increasing the comfortability for any user. Smart HVAC systems are also responsible for the detection of any kind of fault or gradual increment in energy consumption to maintain the conditions of working [30].

Smart Grid: Smart Power Grid Management

Basically, the grid is an electrical network which serves various businesses, residents, and infrastructures in any city. "Smart Grid" is one step ahead of these energy systems, comprising communication technologies and connectivity for the usage of resources in a smart manner. The major components of smart grid are sensors, gateways, radio modules, and routers providing communication and connectivity which results in better consumer energy usage decisions, and cost reduction, enabling authorities for making the system more fault-tolerant, i.e., restoration is easy after blackouts. Various IoT sensors can help in maintaining the street lights to adjust on and off time and management of brightness levels as per real-time conditions which save customer time as well as energy conservation is done to a great extent. Many problem solutions can be done remotely where technicians can troubleshoot the issues remotely and can decide whether physical human presence is required or not [31–33]. Major benefits observed with the application of smart grid are in

- Enabling renewable rnergy generation;
- Better prediction with better billing;
- More resilient.

Smart grid enables the two-way communication within an electric grid making it more resilient, efficient, and green which benefits the consumer, the environment, and the utility company. Thousands of miles of cables can be replaced with wireless technology which makes a great place for smart grids application with its capability to do smart power management.

Smart Agriculture

Individuals are dependent on farmers for daily food, and without it, human survival is not possible making it one of the important sectors where IoT needs to be applied with a promising future. There are various tools developed for crop patterns understanding, distribution of water, and drip irrigation; many drones are deployed for surveillance purpose in farms, and in fact, many hybrid crops are generated and monitored with the help of various devices where a specific type of environment is maintained for that crop to grow [34]. IoT has proven to be of great help to farmers which helps them yielding more productive crops and different types of crops with good management and care perspective.

Smart Healthcare: Telemedicine

One of the popular sayings is "Health is Wealth", and this has been proven to be true in today's world. One of the major applications of IoT in health care is where a sensor is deployed on human body and data is gathered which can predict the disease in the human body. In that case, one can be a part of the assisted living facility, a primary or community health center, an outpatient clinic, or a daycare center all patients can take an advantage of this facility [35]. Another application is where all the previous records and data and testing data are stored in the system about a patient with the help of that all previous records can help in predictions of disease where human body is more vulnerable and can help in decision-making process. For senior citizens, this has proven to be of great usage as remote monitoring can be done via an app, in pandemic, government launched the self-assessment portal for COVID-19 practices and detection on basic level. Many applications are available in market which keep track of human activity such as exercise, breathing, oxygen level, etc., for wellness purpose. These solutions can help in short-term care, preventive care, home care as well as chronic disease management [36].

Smart Shopping

E-commerce has been widely popular for many years, but during the pandemic, it has enhanced its popularity due to people avoiding contact and staying at home following the norms has motivated everyone to do online shopping which has also generated the concept of smart shopping. An automated retail shop has opened in Taiwan where all the products are displayed on an LCD screen and from that LCD screen when selected they will be added to the cart and the bill will be automatically deducted from the user account which is operating with zero human presence. Another example of this is that if a person doesn't want to try the clothing, then they can stand in front of a screen and how that dress or clothing is going to look will be visible on that screen reducing the human effort as well saving the time by a virtual display. Also, with the IoT and artificial intelligence (AI) many brands promote their products in the market virtually with the target audience in mind. Also, the more a person searches about any product on their device the more such kinds of ads are visible to them on their social media handles which is a customizable market advertisement for user needs [37].

Smart Wearables

In the market today, everyone is talking about various types of wearable devices which are put on the human body and its vitals are observed for fitness, medical or wellness purposes. Everyone nowadays is concerned about their health and many IoT startups are working in this field such as Jawbone, which is second to none if we talk about funding. Many new ideas are also proposed in this field where a sensor is deployed in shoe or shirt collar which can help in the achievement of human vitals from different perspectives [38]. Many devices developed in this are now even water protected which can help many sports players such as swimmers to track down their performance and can help in performance evaluation. It can also be helpful to many other sports players as well as common people where vitals can be tracked down for performance evaluation purposes. Still, this field has attracted a lot of researchers as still many improvements and new work need to be done in this field. Some of the major game players in this field are Apple, Fitbit, Pebble, Garmin, Samsung, Huawei, LG, Sony, Microsoft, etc., who are working actively in this field to add utility and drive user management [39].

Smart Industry

Normally, we hear a word known as Industry 4.0 which is one kind of synonym for smart industry and it can be defined as fully integrated and collaborative manner of manufacturing system which responds correspondingly to the demands which keep on changing as well as remains unaffected with the variable conditions in smart industry and meets the customer needs. Smart is virtually connected with IoT, and nowadays, it is popularly also called Industry 4.0; this includes advanced analytics, machine learning (ML), and big data and AI concepts. In the current age, data is the new oil and this concept is based on how an industry can turn data into value and actions where IoT helps a lot in the industries. However, anything which is smart is supposed to serve a purpose otherwise it is of no use that is why industrial internet, Industry 4.0, or industrial IoT are some of the common words which are used for Smart Industry applications. These concepts are widely applied in the field of additive manufacturing, autonomous robots, big data, system integration, cloud computing, IoT, augmented reality, and cybersecurity [40].

Smart Supply-Chain Management

This is also a part of Smart Industry, but one of the main applications of it motivated the author to discuss this in detail separately. With the digital transformation of industry manufacturing processes and its various methods, some of the intermediaries are customization as per mass demands, flexibility in manufacturing, and automation. All these intermediaries exist from raw material to the production of finished goods which include the distributors, retailers, end customers, and wholesalers [41]. Today, many applications have provided a feature that goods are directly sold to customers which includes customized goods as well, e.g., sports equipment. This complete manufacturing system consists of logistic partners, suppliers, manufacturers and partners, and customers. New business models are developed which are based on revenue sources services and data are transforming this complete business chain which has truly become a part of the overall smart supply chain management process to achieve optimization and automation goals.

Smart Military Applications

Military services are back and bone of any nation without whom a nation can stand on its feet peacefully. Technology has proven to be of great help to various organizations, and especially the military, were to prevent human loss drones have proven to be of great help who can fight on human behalf and kill the enemy after deployment. In fact, just like smart cities, military researchers are developing a 'smart base' which contains various modern networks, sensors with enterprise systems for optimization of response times, and decision-making in real-time services. IoT works hand in hand with AI and ML and infrastructures, which are cloud-based, play a pivotal role in the development of Smart Base. Major limitation in developing applications for the military is "Location" because locations are sometimes in such remote areas where no internet or cellular network connections are available. GISinc is one of the major team players in this field who is working continuously with technology changes, location data, and smart bases and developing solutions for smart bases [42] (Table 10.1).

Greening IoT with Fog

As of now, there is a sudden increase in the number of devices. This results in a huge increase in the data. IoT sensor devices which are commonly used by many people are the primary source of data collection. They collect the data in many applications which is also done on the local network side. To accomplish this, a new concept is introduced which is edge/fog computing for the purpose of IoT-based

Table 10.1 Smart applications areas with their components

S. No.	Application area	Smart area	IoT architecture components	Popular applications
1	Consumer application	Smart home	Sensors, protocols, gateways, firmware, databases, middleware, and computing platforms such as cloud computing, fog computing	• Intelligent utility system • Intelligent entertainment • Intelligent electricity meter for water usage • Smart home security having advanced locking system • Smart light/automatic illumination system • Smart surveillance system
2	Infrastructure application	Smart city	Objects, gateways, cloud data, and software applications	• Traffic management • Waste management • Electricity management • Distribution of water
3	Organizational application	Smart transportation	Sensors, actuators, vehicle to vehicle, vehicle to sensor, vehicle to user, vehicle to infrastructure communication, mobile network, GPS	• Smart parking system • Self-driven cars • Smart vehicular management • Accident prevention
4	Infrastructure application	Smart building climate control	Sensors such as humidity, occupancy, temperature, chiller status sensor, connecting medium such as Wi-Fi, Bluetooth, cloud connection	• Smart energy management • Smartly cutting off expenses without human problem • Smart employee experience • Smart space management • Smart portfolio strategy

(continued)

Table 10.1 (continued)

S. No.	Application area	Smart area	IoT architecture components	Popular applications
5	Infrastructure application	Smart grid, smart power grid management	Sensors, gateways, radio modules, and routers	• Renewable energy generation • Billing and predictions • Fault-tolerant • Customer power management
6	Industrial application	Smart agriculture	Sensor technology such as temperature, humidity and wireless sensor nodes, gateway nodes, software application, cellular communication, remote user, database and server	• Crop patterns understanding • Drip irrigation • Water distribution • Tools generation and management • Drones for surveillance • Management and care of crops • Hybrid crop generation
7	Organizational application	Smart healthcare, telemedicine	On-body sensor vitro or vivo sensor, medical device, connecting technology, system management, applications, and end-users	• Tracking wellness of human body • Remote monitoring of patients • Telemedicine • Preventive, self, home care for different age groups
8	Product digitization	Smart shopping	RFID tag, RFID RC reader, Arduino UNO, Bluetooth, server, sensor, management system	• User need-based advertisement • Online virtual trial of products • Offline virtual trial of products
9	Organizational application	Smart wearables	Communication medium, equipment sensor, on-body sensor, gateway, mobile devices	• Health management goals • Fitness/wellness management • Drive user management • Performance evaluation

(continued)

Table 10.1 (continued)

S. No.	Application area	Smart area	IoT architecture components	Popular applications
10	Industrial applications	Smart industry	Gateway, sensor, application models, control applications, device administration, user administration, and security monitoring	• Meet user needs • Produce products efficiently • Reduction in human efforts • Tracking and management of resources
11	Industrial applications	Smart supply-chain management	Sensor, gateways, tracking of real-time location, condition status, and exception alerts such as delays and network medium such as GSM, WiFi, etc.	• Management of flow of product • Management of flow of information
12	Military applications	Smart military	Sensor, CCTV, gateway, RFID, LTE connection, GPS, drones, data access, storage, and distribution medium	• Smart base • Drone deployment for prevention of human life loss • Smart amination

applications. Initially, these requests were processed on cloud due to the availability of high computational resources. But as resources are being utilized, it becomes overwhelming leading to a need to decrease the load on the cloud. Now, a new concept which is fog computing is used so that the requests which are sent by IoT sensing devices are first processed on the fog layer. If the requested resources are available on the fog itself, then an immediate response will be provided. If in case of unavailability, a request will be made to the cloud. Efficient results have been observed in many applications when fog computing is used in place of cloud layer. Though fog can't be a complete replacement for the cloud at any point of time. Currently, there is a lot of research going on in the field of scalability, resource management, security improvement, mobility, etc., many researchers can address these fields of applications for their further research goals [43]. Generally, when we talk about fog computing, it provides three kinds of services in greening IoT which are discussed as follows and addressed in Fig. 10.2:

- Computing Services: Cloud architecture follows the processing where tasks are processed on the cloud to fog for less time consumption and processing on local level. This brings to the concept of different processing requirements as compared to the actual work. To understand this better, we can take an example of pattern recognition where distribution of resources needs to be done in such a way that frequently used patterns should be located at the fog layer and general patterns can

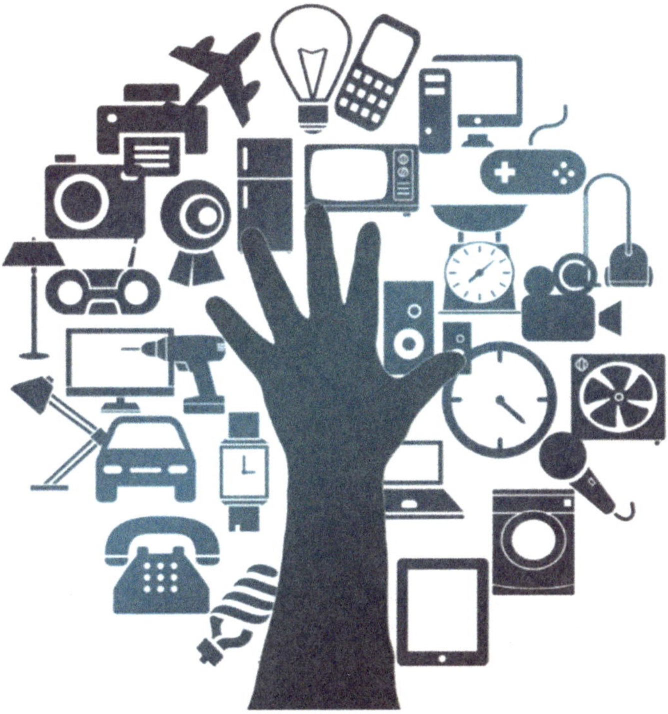

Fig. 10.2 IoT applications and enabling technologies [44]

be made available in the cloud as they are not of frequent usage. These services help in the improvement of reliability of the whole system as management of data can be done and responses to the events can be handled in real-time applications.

- Communication Services: There is always an issue with resources in the smart layers in devices. Communication is controlled by wireless protocols in IoT architecture. These protocols are helpful in efficient power operations, good coverage, and narrowband transmissions. Placement of the fog layer is done in such a way that communication is combined together and done into a single communication which is further used by clouds. This also results in the enhancement of reliability of the overall system.
- Storage Services: IoT architecture includes an unlimited number of devices which results in a huge amount of data generation. One limitation here is that devices are with very less storage capabilities. One of the options here is to transfer the data to the cloud, but due to high demand in the cloud despite having high computational capabilities and storage capabilities, it arises an issue. Therefore, an urge comes to temporary storage of data in fog. In this type of service, they can compress, analyze, and filter the data with the learning of information available locally. As end devices are not having storage capabilities and also communication is not that

robust, here this service can help in providing an improved system behavior and hence enhancing the reliability of the system.

Protocols with Enabling Technologies

There are many protocols with the technologies for deployment of effective fog–IoT–cloud-based systems. There is a need to explore the methods with which we can make communication effective in the IoT-based system. Some of these enabling technologies and protocols which improve the interoperability in the topologies, applications, and technologies are as follows:

- RFID: They operate at a 125 kHz frequency band. Their requirement is a 12 V supply of power. They are composed of readers and tags. Their principal work is to reflect the radio wave back and pass it further to the readers.
- WISP: This is a wireless and battery-free platform used for computation and sensing purposes. They use ultra-high-frequency RFID readers.
- WSN: This can be easily integrated with the existing IoT architecture. Many researchers have worked in this field and they have found out that world sensors can be deployed to monitor appliances in sustainable smart cities.
- BLE: This technology operates at a 2.4 GHz frequency band. It can be easily amalgamated into Bluetooth technology and provides benefits. Many applications where it can be deployed are monitoring purposes in medical and industrial situations and transportation systems.
- NFC: This method operated at a 13.56 MHz frequency. Simple devices such as cards and stickers are targeted which allows devices to communicate in P2P manner when both the devices that want to communicate are powered.
- IEEE: Many protocols such as IEEE802.11ah and 802.15.4 standards are followed. When we talk in congested networks, protocol IEEE802.11ah outperforms with less energy consumption.
- Z-Wave: This is a MAC protocol operating at a 908 MHz frequency with less power consumption. It operates at a low data rate making it unsuitable to use in time-sensitive critical applications.
- LTE-A: This is an extension of the LTE network. Lower latencies and higher throughput are provided with good coverage. Its multi-antenna feature makes it suitable for using in fog-based structures.
- LoRaWAN: This is basically a low-power wide-area network technology supporting long-range operations with less power consumption and less rate of data. With the usage of a single hop, IoT devices can communicate with gateways in fog–IoT architecture making it of utmost importance.
- IPv6: This protocol provides an enhancement over IPv4 by providing a unique address to each IoT device. It supports IPSec protocol for security.
- 6LoWPAN: This is a network protocol which operates at 2.4 GHz with low power capabilities. It helps in enabling IPv6 to operate with low power transmission capabilities.

- NB-IOT: This is a less power-consuming technology which is typically designed for IoT coverage. It is helpful in connection with objects requiring data of small amounts and for a longer duration. This technology is being deployed in various smart city applications such as smart hospitals and smart parking systems. This protocol helps in bandwidth usage reduction by maintaining a good quality of analysis of data with efficient response time and data storage capabilities.
- SigFox: This is a network protocol which provides M2MWAN communication. The band at which it operates is 868 MHz frequency. This is helpful in reduction of cost, improvement in range of communication, enhancement in capacity of network, and life cycle enhancement of the device.

IoT and Fog with Other Technologies Working Towards Sustainability

Recently, due to an increase in the number of devices, there is an urge to meet the computational demands in real-time application-based scenarios. This brings fog computing into the picture as it provides computation capabilities near to the end-user. Resultant to which is reduction in time delays and improvement in latency-sensitive applications. Moreover, many other technologies are working hand in hand such as AI and ML in fog-IoT-based architecture. To work towards sustainable smart cities, there is a huge potential to discuss such technologies. For a few of these organizations, in real-time applications, data measurement deploys the AI- and ML-based model to impact the initiatives taken towards sustainability like [43].

Oil and Gas organizations are deploying edge technologies for monitoring purposes. They try to monitor the health of stack flare and understand the output emissions. Edge solutions when infused with sensor technology can be of great help such as it can help in the identification of compressor health issues and can also be very helpful in alerting regarding regulatory violations.

Steel manufacturers are also deploying edge-based solutions for the prevention of CO2 transmissions. It is also helpful in the identification of any part produced which is defective in nature in the early stage. This can be further helpful in increasing yield and help in the reduction of scraps.

Many transportation organizations are considering to deploy edge-based solutions by using and driving green technology which can help in detection and reduction of emission of huge amounts of CO2 emissions which are happening every year [44].

Conclusion

The IoT has emerged a lot in this era, and with its technological advancements, everybody has seen its usage and power. Now, we all know that all the applications of research are based on the concept of how to make it smarter and more adaptable to society, which further arises the term "Smart is the New Green". In this chapter, we have thoroughly discussed various smart applications such as smart homes, smart buildings, smart grids, smart transportation, etc. From a researcher's point of view, it has attracted us a lot to learn about the emerging technologies with the network protocol which are used in the communication of IoT devices. In smart city architecture, end devices rely to pass the collected data and query to be processed on cloud. Due to huge demand and lack of ability of cloud to meet those demands, a new concept arises which is fog computing. Here in this chapter, we have discussed how IoT and fog can work hand in hand towards sustainability. Also, edge-based solutions are collaborating with other technologies to provide solutions in the current era. From a researcher' perspective, this topic has withdrawn our interest and a lot of potentials is found where still research gaps are there and are required to be addressed such as management of resources, efficient energy consumption, security protocols, etc.

References

1. Zahmatkesh, H., Al-, F.: Fog computing for sustainable smart cities in the IoT era: caching techniques and enabling technologies-an overview. Sustain. Cities Soc. **59**, 102139 (2020)
2. Subbarao, V., Srinivas, K., Pavithr, R.S.: A survey on internet of things based smart, digital green and intelligent campus. In: 2019 4th International Conference on Internet of Things: Smart Innovation and Usages (IoT-SIU), pp. 1–6. IEEE (2019, April)
3. Jalali, F., Khodadustan, S., Gray, C., Hinton, K., Suits, F.: Greening iot with fog: a survey. In: 2017 IEEE International Conference on Edge Computing (EDGE), pp. 25–31. IEEE (2017, June)
4. Su, K., Li, J., Fu, H.: Smart city and the applications. In: 2011 International Conference on Electronics, Communications and Control (ICECC), pp. 1028–1031. IEEE (2011, September)
5. Bakıcı, T., Almirall, E., Wareham, J.: A smart city initiative: the case of Barcelona. J. Knowl. Econ. **4**(2), 135–148 (2013)
6. Hall, R.E., Bowerman, B., Braverman, J., Taylor, J., Todosow, H., Von Wimmersperg, U.: The vision of a smart city. No. BNL-67902; 04042, Brookhaven National Lab., Upton, NY (US) (2000)
7. Shelton, T., Zook, M., Wiig, A.: The 'actually existing smart city.' Camb. J. Reg. Econ. Soc. **8**(1), 13–25 (2015)
8. Vanolo, A.: Smartmentality: the smart city as disciplinary strategy. Urban Stud. **51**(5), 883–898 (2014)
9. Nam, T., Pardo, T.A.: Conceptualizing smart city with dimensions of technology, people, and institutions. In: Proceedings of the 12th Annual International Digital Government Research Conference: Digital Government Innovation in Challenging Times, pp. 282–291 (2011, June)
10. Dameri, R.P.: Searching for smart city definition: a comprehensive proposal. Int. J. Comput. Technol. **11**(5), 2544–2551 (2013)
11. Neirotti, P., De Marco, A., Cagliano, A.C., Mangano, G., Scorrano, F.: Current trends in smart city initiatives: some stylised facts. Cities **38**, 25–36 (2014)
12. Angelidou, M.: Smart city policies: a spatial approach. Cities **41**, S3–S11 (2014)
13. Kim, T.H., Ramos, C., Mohammed, S.: Smart city and IoT (2017)
14. Gaur, A., Scotney, B., Parr, G., McClean, S.: Smart city architecture and its applications based on IoT. Procedia Comput. Sci. **52**, 1089–1094 (2015)
15. Theodoridis, E., Mylonas, G., Chatzigiannakis, I.: Developing an iot smart city framework. In: IISA 2013, pp. 1–6. IEEE (2013, July)

16. Datta, P., Sharma, B.: A survey on IoT architectures, protocols, security and smart city based applications. In: 2017 8th International Conference on Computing, Communication and Networking Technologies (ICCCNT), pp. 1–5. IEEE (2017, July)
17. Sterbenz, J.P.: Smart city and IoT resilience, survivability, and disruption tolerance: challenges, modelling, and a survey of research opportunities. In: 2017 9th International Workshop on Resilient Networks Design and Modeling (RNDM), pp. 1–6. IEEE (2017, September)
18. Byun, J., Kim, S., Sa, J., Kim, S., Shin, Y.T., Kim, J.B.: Smart city implementation models based on IoT technology. Adv. Sci. Technol. Lett. **129**(41), 209–212 (2016)
19. Bounceur, A.: CupCarbon: a new platform for designing and simulating smart-city and IoT wireless sensor networks (SCI-WSN). In: Proceedings of the International Conference on Internet of things and Cloud Computing, p. 1 (2016, March)
20. Mishra, S.K., Puthal, D., Rodrigues, J.J., Sahoo, B., Dutkiewicz, E.: Sustainable service allocation using a metaheuristic technique in a fog server for industrial applications. IEEE Trans. Ind. Inf. **14**(10), 4497–4506 (2018)
21. Puthal, D., Obaidat, M.S., Nanda, P., Prasad, M., Mohanty, S.P., Zomaya, A.Y.: Secure and sustainable load balancing of edge data centers in fog computing. IEEE Commun. Mag. **56**(5), 60–65 (2018)
22. Wallace, T., Gibbons, D., O'Dwyer, M., Curran, T.P.: International evolution of fat, oil and grease (FOG) waste management–a review. J. Environ. Manage. **187**, 424–435 (2017)
23. Rahman, M.A., Hossain, M.S., Hassanain, E., Muhammad, G.: Semantic multimedia fog computing and IoT environment: sustainability perspective. IEEE Commun. Mag. **56**(5), 80–87 (2018)
24. Bratina, B., Šorgo, A., Kramberger, J., Ajdnik, U., Zemljič, L.F., Ekart, J., Šafarič, R.: From municipal/industrial wastewater sludge and FOG to fertilizer: a proposal for economic sustainable sludge management. J. Environ. Manage. **183**, 1009–1025 (2016)
25. Verma, S., Yadav, A.K., Motwani, D., Raw, R.S., Singh, H.K.: An efficient data replication and load balancing technique for fog computing environment. In: 2016 3rd International Conference on Computing for Sustainable Global Development (INDIACom), pp. 2888–2895. IEEE (2016, March)
26. Kaur, J., Agrawal, A., Khan, R.A.: Security issues in fog environment: a systematic literature review. Int. J. Wirel. Inf. Netw. **27**, 467–483 (2020)
27. Adhikari, M., Gianey, H.: Energy efficient offloading strategy in fog-cloud environment for IoT applications. Internet Things **6**, 100053 (2019)
28. Dutta, J., Roy, S.: IoT-fog-cloud based architecture for smart city: prototype of a smart building. In: 2017 7th International Conference on Cloud Computing, Data Science & Engineering-Confluence, pp. 237–242. IEEE (2017, January)
29. Mohamed, N., Al-Jaroodi, J., Jawhar, I.: Towards fault tolerant fog computing for IoT-based smart city applications. In 2019 IEEE 9th Annual Computing and Communication Workshop and Conference (CCWC), pp. 0752–0757. IEEE (2019, January)
30. Naranjo, P.G.V., Pooranian, Z., Shojafar, M., Conti, M., Buyya, R.: FOCAN: A Fog-supported smart city network architecture for management of applications in the Internet of Everything environments. J. Parallel Distrib. Comput. **132**, 274–283 (2019)
31. Alli, A.A., Alam, M.M.: SecOFF-FCIoT: machine learning based secure offloading in Fog-Cloud of things for smart city applications. Internet Things **7**, 100070 (2019)
32. Mohamed, N., Al-, J., Jawhar, I., Lazarova, S., Mahmoud, S.: SmartCityWare: a service-oriented middleware for cloud and fog enabled smart city services. IEEE Access **5**, 17576–17588 (2017)
33. Wang, T., Liang, Y., Jia, W., Arif, M., Liu, A., Xie, M.: Coupling resource management based on fog computing in smart city systems. J. Netw. Comput. Appl. **135**, 11–19 (2019)
34. Bruneo, D., Distefano, S., Longo, F., Merlino, G., Puliafito, A., D'Amico, V., Torrisi, G.: Stack4Things as a fog computing platform for smart city applications. In: 2016 IEEE Conference on Computer Communications Workshops (INFOCOM WKSHPS), pp. 848–853. IEEE (2016, April)

35. Zhang, C.: Design and application of fog computing and Internet of Things service platform for smart city. Futur. Gener. Comput. Syst. **112**, 630–640 (2020)
36. Santos, J., Wauters, T., Volckaert, B., De Turck, F.: Fog computing: enabling the management and orchestration of smart city applications in 5G networks. Entropy **20**(1), 4 (2018)
37. Giordano, A., Spezzano, G., Vinci, A.: Smart agents and fog computing for smart city applications. In: International Conference on Smart Cities, pp. 137–146. Springer, Cham (2016, June)
38. Bellavista, P., Chatzimisios, P., Foschini, L., Paradisioti, M., Scotece, D.: A support infrastructure for machine learning at the edge in smart city surveillance. In: 2019 IEEE Symposium on Computers and Communications (ISCC), pp. 1189–1194. IEEE (2019, June)
39. Chen, N., Chen, Y.: Smart city surveillance at the network edge in the era of iot: opportunities and challenges. In: Smart Cities, pp. 153–176 (2018)
40. Moh, M., Raju, R.: Machine learning techniques for security of Internet of Things (IoT) and fog computing systems. In: 2018 International Conference on High Performance Computing & Simulation (HPCS), pp. 709–715. IEEE (2018, July)
41. Mohammadi, M., Al-, A.: Enabling cognitive smart cities using big data and machine learning: approaches and challenges. IEEE Commun. Mag. **56**(2), 94–101 (2018)
42. Rocha Neto, A.F., Delicato, F.C., Batista, T.V., Pires, P.F.: Distributed machine learning for iot applications in the fog. In: Fog Computing: Theory and Practice, pp. 309–345 (2020)
43. Bhargava, A., Salunkhe, G., Bhargava, S., Goswami, P.: A comprehensive study of IoT security risks in building a secure smart city. In: Digital Cities Roadmap: IoT-Based Architecture and Sustainable Buildings, pp. 401–448 (2021)
44. Rahman, M.A., Rashid, M.M., Hossain, M.S., Hassanain, E., Alhamid, M.F., Guizani, M.: Blockchain and IoT-based cognitive edge framework for sharing economy services in a smart city. IEEE Access **7**, 18611–18621 (2019)

Chapter 11
Role of the Fourth Industrial Revolution Towards Sustainable Development

Rintu Nath

Introduction

During the last decade, we have seen unprecedented growth in technology. Exponential growth in information technology and faster than ever communication speed is changing manufacturing, agriculture, healthcare, education, servicing, and delivery systems. Artificial intelligence-based systems are replacing human labour and supplementing the human decision-making process in a more decisive way. The Fourth Industrial Revolution (4IR) is due to technology breakthroughs in wide-ranging fields such as nanotechnology, biotechnology, AI, robotics, 3D printing, material science, high-performance computing, etc., to name a few [1]. 4IR is leading towards a holistic change in the majority of sectors and society as a whole. New age computing and automation have long-term implications and it has the ability to modify or replace conventional methods of human interference in manufacturing, agriculture, and almost all service sectors. These changes will have overlapping effects on the workforce. It is, therefore, desirable that the 4IR is sustainable, able to narrow the gap between rich and poor, ensures gender equality, and is beneficial for people in general.

4IR will change the entire working systems of manufacturing, agriculture, transportation, and associated processes. Machines have already replaced labour-intensive and repetitive jobs to increase efficiency and higher productivity. This way, 4IR will create more innovative and challenging jobs for human resources. The key is an adaptation to the changes and skill up-gradation with new technologies. 4IR should not be viewed as a conflict between man and machine—competing for sustainability. 4IR-driven automation will create a framework where hi-tech machines will supplement

R. Nath (✉)
Vigyan Prasar, Department of Science and Technology, Technology Bhawan, New Mehrauli Road, New Delhi 110016, India
e-mail: Rnath@vigyanprasar.gov.in

A. Choudhury et al. (eds.), *Evolution of Digitized Societies Through Advanced Technologies*, Advanced Technologies and Societal Change,
https://doi.org/10.1007/978-981-19-2984-7_11

human resources to increase productivity. Coordinated efforts from all stakeholders need to ensure ceaseless integration of new technology with the existing one to generate more jobs.

Drivers of 4IR

Several interconnected developments in ICT and their applications in physical systems are the drivers of 4IR. The increase in powers of computer processors, innovations in communication technology, and the adaptation of distributed computing are primary factors responsible for the information technology boom. Artificial intelligence (AI) based on machine learning (ML) and deep learning (DL) is not only leading machine automation but also able to contribute to cognitive skills. Efficient and smaller sensors can connect products, services, and places with humans. The Internet of Things (IoT) is the result of this connected technology and one of the drivers of 4IR. Combined communications with sensor networks, intelligent real-time processing, embedded systems, and automated operation are also referred to as cyber-physical systems [2]. New materials like graphene and polyhexahydrotriazine (PHT) are contributing to new age smart devices. Graphene is much stronger than steel and also conducts electricity and heat. PHT is thermoset plastic that can be reused. It can be used in mobile phones, circuit boards, and many other products that are not easily recyclable. Another significant contributor to 4IR is 3D printing technology. Although 3D printing is useful for making prototypes, the availability of a new range of materials promises it to be considered a viable option for industrial production. Using 3D printing, both aesthetic and functional models can be created. Some other drivers of 4IR are AI-driven advanced robotics and autonomous vehicles. Increased research in interdisciplinary fields, including computer science and engineering, mechanical, electrical, electronics, and basic sciences, will lead to advanced robotics and associated developments. Self-driven vehicles are going to take a significant role in transportation. Armed with GPS, radar, sonar, and many more measuring and controlling devices, sensors, and transducers, these futuristic vehicles are all set to drive 4IR to a new height.

Technology Trends

During the last decade, information and communication technology could provide solutions to the majority of problems. Solutions provided by ICT are based on data analysis, and in most cases, they are cost-effective [3]. High-speed processors, availability of data, reliable communication link, and efficient data handling models provide opportunities to churn out patterns to understand requirement trends, demand–supply, production, and services. Gap analysis of different workflows is done to increase productivity. Machine learning and deep-learning-enabled models can analyse a large volume of data, generate outputs accurately, and draw inferences, depending on the requirement.

We are in an era where any device and sensor can be accessed and controlled remotely using high-speed internet. Everything can be controlled remotely, from a household lamp, vehicle, machinery to a space shuttle. The estimation is that by 2025, there will be 100 billion devices under the IoT network through a variety of sensors [4]. In other words, most people will be directly or indirectly connected with machines. With 4IR, human-to-machine (H2M) and machine-to-machine (M2M) roles are rapidly evolving.

Automation and Associated Fear of Job Loss

Technology-driven industries will be able to leverage changing trends in automation-based manufacturing: jobs that are repetitive, labour-intensive, and hazardous need to be replaced by robots. Robots can increase productivity many folds with zero error. Manufacturing units across the globe are increasingly relying on process automation to increase efficiency and reduction of manufacturing costs. This, however, has associated risks of job loss, particularly for unskilled or semi-skilled workers. Elimination of jobs is seen as a potential threat across the globe, particularly to developing countries. Professions that are not likely to be affected and most likely to be affected by 4IR are listed in Table 11.1.

Structural job reduction is noticed in many industries across the globe. The maximum impact is generally on semi- and unskilled labourers, who make up a substantial portion of the manufacturing and agricultural sectors. Already, a

Table 11.1 Professions that will be highly affected and least affected by automation

Highly affected by automation	Least affected by automation
Farm labour contractors	Psychologists
Secretaries and administrative assistants, except legal, medical, and executive	Human resource managers
Couriers and messengers	Mental health and substance abuse social workers
Real estate brokers	Choreographers
Hosts and hostesses	Computer systems analysts
Legal secretaries	Sales manager
Umpires, referees and other sports officials	Chief executives
Insurance appraisers, auto damage	Anthropologists and archaeologists
Tax preparers	Physicians and surgeons
Telemarketers	Marine engineers and naval architects

Source Carl Benedikt Frey and Michael Osborne, University of Oxford, 2013

downward trend in compensation towards unskilled and semi-skilled workforce is observed. The International Labour Organization (ILO) has documented [5] the share of unskilled labour compensation in the GDP of different countries. It is seen that the decline in share is more profound in developing countries.

Paradigm Shift

With 4IR, significant changes in types of jobs, availability, and location are expected. Three situations can be envisaged: existing jobs are redefined, machines replace humans, and creation of new jobs [6]. Automation-related job losses may be countered by creating new jobs. A section of these newly created jobs will be required for maintenance of machines and up-gradation to newer technologies. However, these new jobs would demand new skill sets. Continuous upskilling and reskilling are going to be a major driving force to maintain the growth and sustainability of 4IR. Another important factor is the locational displacement of the workforce. Some jobs will be location-independent, while some other jobs would need a considerable shift of location. A large section of the present workforce, like people who are working for agricultural produce or light manufacturing units, would thus be vulnerable due to automation and may have to switch to other types of jobs and associated shifts in location [7]. It is expected that initiatives will be taken by governments and other stakeholders such that new jobs are accessible to these vulnerable groups. 4IR promises new business models and more skill-centred start-up ventures.

The Emergence of New Professions

The effect of 4IR is going to be in every sphere of our life, including employment. The future of repetitive, unskilled jobs is a cause of significant concern. There is no denying that a change is on its way, and there will be a significant impact on the labour market and workplaces worldwide. However, this change should not be viewed as a machine-versus-man dilemma. Connected technology will enable enhanced skill sets with better cognition [8]. Upskilling and reskilling of human resources will develop a new ecosystem that can work alongside AI-driven machines.

Fill the Gap

It is required to map the competence and skill set expected by different industries in the next 5 years and 10 years horizon. Demand for skills that enable the adaptation of new technologies will increase many folds. Some areas that are not fully covered by automation, like psychological health assessment and human resource manager, as mentioned in Table 11.1, will need more human resources to fill the gap. There is a possibility of the non-availability of a skilled workforce that may limit innovation and growth [9].

Gender Equality

New positions and professions will emerge due to 4IR. In addition, non-technological factors like socio-political interference and new cultural norms will contribute to this change [10]. We should take full advantage of 4IR to ensure that women and men are equally empowered in the coming years.

Social Equality

4IR is technology-driven and expected to improve the quality of life in general. With skill up-gradation, people will be more productive. As the economy improves, the benefit can be returned to people with higher remuneration and better perks [9]. 4IR is also expected to remove social and gender biases. In general, labour-intensive jobs are male-dominated. With paradigm shifts, technology-driven jobs will not have such biases.

Challenges

More and more people must be able to harness benefits from 4IR. Increasing efficiency through automation and related job reduction may adversely affect some sections, and long-term growth may be stalled. A holistic framework that empowers people from all sections to adapt to changing job requirements with a new set of skills can only be sustainable. While investing to develop new technologies is essential, its impact on existing scenarios should also be assessed. Technology innovation without skill up-gradation will lead to the non-availability of required human resources [11]. For example, introducing a new machine in an assembly line of a manufacturing unit will lead to production loss if adequate training is not provided to the people who handle it. Hence investment towards skill up-gradation will be very important.

There is surging unemployment globally across all industries. An innovative framework for new business models is required to reduce unemployment. Otherwise, a consumer demand reduction will lead to a weaker economy, and a vicious cycle would start [12]. Unfortunately, many manufacturers feel that technology-driven automation and workers are two opposite sides; only one can survive. Developing a mutually dependent relationship where technology can extend workers' capability towards increased efficiency and growth is one of the significant challenges of 4IR.

Conclusion

It is required to investigate how technology-enabled manufacturing and associated industries will change business opportunities and employment. Effects on the manufacturer, consumers, and other stakeholders need to be assessed. Government-funded institutions need to focus on skill up-gradation, especially for unskilled and semi-skilled workforces. Data analysis can be done to understand how 4IR is changing manufacturing processes, creating jobs, and improving the overall well-being of workers. We do not yet fully understand how technology will unfold in terms of complexity, interconnections of human to machine (H2M), machine to machine (M2M), and adaptation among all stakeholders. It is, however, imperative that a shared understanding is crucial for a collective future to ensure equality in sharing knowledge and resources, reducing the gap between poor and rich, and extending benefits to all in general. Technology-driven 4IR needs to be human-centric to transform the entire system for a better and sustainable future that can be extended across countries and societies.

References

1. Schwab, K.: The Fourth Industrial Revolution. World Economic Forum, Geneva (2016)
2. Summit, M., Moavenzadeh, J., Forum, W.E.: The 4th Industrial Revolution -Reshaping the Future of Production. World Economic Forum, Geneva (2015)
3. Bagnoli, C., Dal Mas, F., Massaro, M.: The 4th industrial revolution: business models and evidence from the field. Int. J. E-Serv. Mob. Appl. **11**(3), 34–47 (2019). https://doi.org/10.4018/IJESMA.2019070103
4. Taylor, R., Baron, D., Schmidt, D.: The world in 2025 - predictions for the next ten years. In: 10th International Microsystems, Packaging, Assembly and Circuits Technology Conference (IMPACT 2015) - Proceedings, pp. 192–195 (2015). https://doi.org/10.1109/IMPACT.2015.7365193
5. OECD: The labour share in G20 economies. Report prepared for the G20 Employment Working Group, February, pp. 1–22 (2015)
6. Skilton, M., Hovsepian, F.: Mastering the 4th Industrial Revolution (2016)
7. Kodama, F.: Learning mode and strategic concept for the 4th industrial revolution. J. Open Innov. Technol. Mark. Complex. **4**(3), 32 (2018). https://doi.org/10.3390/joitmc4030032
8. Spöttl, G., Windelband, L.: The 4th industrial revolution–its impact on vocational skills. J. Educ. Work **34**(1), 29–52 (2021). https://doi.org/10.1080/13639080.2020.1858230
9. Pitsis, T.S., Beckman, S.L., Steinert, M., Oviedo, L., Maisch, B.: Designing the future: strategy, design, and the 4th industrial revolution—an introduction to the special issue. Calif. Manage. Rev. **62**(2), 5–11 (2020). https://doi.org/10.1177/0008125620907163
10. Leurent, H., Betti, F., Shook, E., Fuchs, R., Damrath, F.: Leading through the fourth industrial revolution - putting people at the centre. World Economic Forum, January, pp. 1–25 (2019)

11. Oke, A., Fernandes, F.A.P.: Innovations in teaching and learning - exploring the perceptions of the education sector on the 4th industrial revolution (4IR). J. Open Innov. Technol. Mark. Complex. **6**(2), 31 (2020). https://doi.org/10.3390/JOITMC6020031
12. Pereira Pessôa, M.V., Jauregui Becker, J.M.: Smart design engineering: a literature review of the impact of the 4th industrial revolution on product design and development. Res. Eng. Des. **31**(2), 175–195 (2020). https://doi.org/10.1007/s00163-020-00330-z

Chapter 12
An Extensive Framework Focused on Smart Agriculture Based Out of IoT

Manish Thakral, Rishi Raj Singh, and Sandeep Pratap Singh

Introduction

By the year 2102, the Central Statistical Division estimates the world population will rise to about 10.9 billion [1]. There is an increasing need for agriculture to enhance crop yields safely as the world rapidly increases. Feeding people and protecting the environment both help people and save natural resources. The resultant interest in food and agricultural markets has expanded to include politicians, international donors, nongovernmental organisations, and commercial companies. Agriculture is currently undergoing radical transformations and must also deal with various environmental and social issues. Traditional agricultural techniques are still in use by many farmers who have little market access, and balancing the demands on natural resources like land has proven challenging. Although dietary changes, as well as consumer preferences, and the issue of climate change all play a role in helping to provide higher-quality food to the customer, these changes and causes only contribute to the total complexity of food services [2]. With the current agricultural techniques that have led to considerable deforestation, water shortages, or water pollution, healthy forestry and medical production are not possible. In order to provide a more sustainable basis for natural resources, sophisticated methods are employed which preserve and enhance the basis of natural resources and improve productivity. "Comprehensive" approaches go through a process of time similar to smart agriculture [3]. A smart approach to farming guidance that takes into account climate change is available. In 2008, the concept of smart agriculture initially appeared and later gained momentum as several stakeholders actively engaged in the process of

M. Thakral (✉) · R. R. Singh · S. P. Singh
School of Computer Science, UPES, Dehradun, India
e-mail: Manishthakra@gmail.com

S. P. Singh
e-mail: spsingh@ddn.upes.ac.in

A. Choudhury et al. (eds.), *Evolution of Digitized Societies Through Advanced Technologies*, Advanced Technologies and Societal Change,
https://doi.org/10.1007/978-981-19-2984-7_12

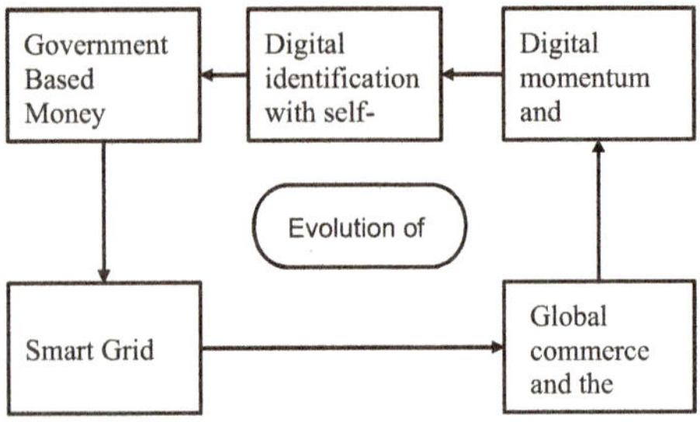

Fig. 12.1 Illustration of blockchain prediction with IoT standard

formulation and construction. Many of the key aspects of the best farming concept have been created in light of the ongoing debates on agricultural policy, as a way to advance sustainable growth [4]. Figure 12.1 depicts the evolution of technology. Climate change mitigation and rural food production may be addressed using smart agriculture practices. Data collection, data analysis, and data presentation are all involved in precision agriculture. Smart agriculture uses advanced transformation methods such as Internet of Things, business intelligence, and cloud technology to collect data, analyse data, and make information available to farmers so they can make informed decisions [5].

Farming Using IoT

Internet of Things (IoT) is a groundbreaking platform that incorporates slicing computer and networking concepts. Throughout the future, intelligent technology will be about Internet of Things. Many computer systems at home and in the office are being transformed by the introduction of Internet of Things (IoT). Internet of Things (IoT) uses a network of connected computers or nodes to provide multimedia services to other systems. By linking billions of devices to the Internet, Internet of Things (IoT) holds tremendous promise for smart objects [6]. Smart objects are equipped with sensors that are capable of gathering data and networking with other devices over the Internet. As Internet of Things (IoT) has grown, the technology has advanced to the next level, bringing numerous farming possibilities [7]. IoT enables a broad spectrum of applications in the area of smart farming, such as soil and plant tracking, inspection of crop growth and choosing, support for watering management, and development of agriculture. Diagnosis and control technologies are used in intelligent agriculture [8]. The field application of IoT has enhanced the productivity and efficiency of farmers in order to maximise agriculture. It can contribute to determining field factors such as soil and plant growth. It may also be used for testing and monitoring factors such as heat, soil humidity, and crop illness. IoT may also be used to track the influencing elements in agricultural development and production. Growers are also able to find which plants are most suitable and may rotate the crop accordingly. In phosphorus fertiliser, watering, processing of crops,

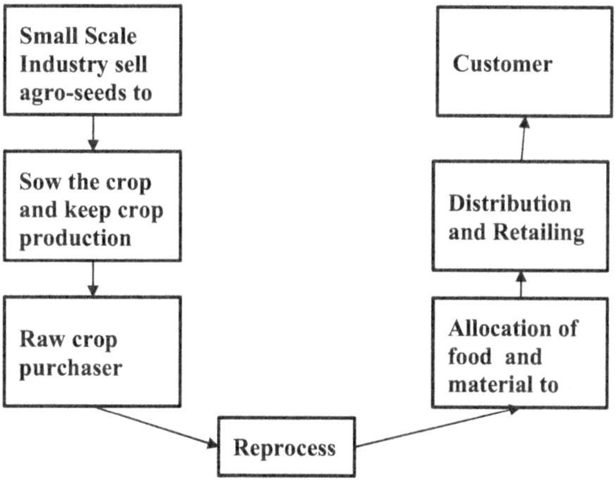

Fig. 12.2 Management of food chain

reaping and post-harvesting, storage of crops and transit, and many more benefits in agricultural IoT systems, IoT applications help farmers [9].

Food Management System

The management of the food system is a procedure that describes how foodstuffs from a farm end up on our plates. Management of the supply chain deals with the manufacture, processing, distribution, sales, evacuation, and consumption [10]. The supply procedure sums up the chain. In the developing world, there are several problems in the food system, such as the requirement for trust amongst suppliers frequently linked to their creditworthiness and accountability. Users of the product and risk management difficulties, delays, or disorders are often caused by inadequate or lack of information. Blockchain is one of the finest technologies to resolve this issue [11]. Figure 12.2 depicts how the management of food works.

Blockchain Enables IoT

Blockchain A database is a collection of data that may be saved, exchanged, and secured via a decentralised computer network, but only the proprietor with a unique number may perform transactions if the information is disseminated. Participating nodes are other machines or computers on the network. Transactions between nodes are reliably recorded in a public directory without the help of a trusted person [12]. In a centralised cloud method, an asset or item is the property of a public authority, such as a bank, or it is owned by an owner. There is always one server for multiple clients for a centralised computer system; there is greater capacity for the server than its application servers and every operation is done by a single server, which is now a conventional technique [13]. Blockchain stores block unit operations, and each block includes brick background hashes, blockchain pots, time, relevant information, and block purchases. When a transmitter node creates a trade, it transfers it to other network nodes. The receiver networks check the event and have evidence. The successful node will transmit it to all the other peers and join the block with the blockchain. The operation must be confirmed by an originator and contain the key to encrypting a message. Some other nodes will thus check the transaction's legitimacy. The hash of the preceding block is included in each block, which indicates that every block is connected [14]. It may help build trust in the agriculture supply chains by using reliable data connecting supply chain participants. Food items all the way from the farm to the grocery store became a reality [15]. Food system real-time surveillance and detection of actual sources are significant benefits of using blockchain and IoT. It makes it easier to identify the most prominent Nike supply chain [16]. Farmers, like their peers in the agricultural sector, often use potentially harmful pesticides in order to increase crop yields and yield per acre. Second, there is an increase in food frauds and incorrect statistical data [17].

Blockchain is a technology that was developed for the agricultural industry, and it is now being used in the production process to establish a new supply chain for the agricultural sector. There is a repository that maintains track of and organises all of the paper-based documentation that is created. There are also material and economic aspects to take into account. Because of the implementation of blockchain technology, it is possible that both accountability and the quality of payments will increase. With its capacity to compete for processes and transactions throughout the agricultural supply chain in real time, this cutting-edge technology has the potential to disrupt the whole agricultural supply chain. It is currently undergoing beta testing. Every contact in the natural world has a major impact. When product-specific features and transactions are incorporated into the product's design, this is referred to as dissemination. Investigation and discovery of linkages between commodities at all levels of the supply chain, as well as relationships between items at various points in the supply chain, are required. They practise fertilisers in combination with other companies, such as fertiliser, feeding, and medical clinics, in order to maximise their profits [18]. Furthermore, unlike traditional databases, Blockchain retains records that are both open and incorruptible, making it a superior alternative to traditional databases. It is also accessible to any supply chain partners who have a digital presence, in addition to the general public. These technological advancements provide the opportunity to achieve huge efficiency while also delivering possible benefits to each individual member of the organisation. Blockchain provides a platform for accountability in the food supply chain, allowing customers to track the items they purchase all the way back to the farm and guarantee that they are of the highest possible quality throughout the process. authenticity. Tracing the movement of a product makes it simpler to pursue legal responsibility for copyright infringement, which in turn makes it easier to put in place regulatory measures to protect consumers. It is maintained by the use of blockchain technology, which is a distributed ledger [19].

Integration of IoT with Industry

A wonderful innovation, Internet of Things (IoT) is a crucial participant in the technological revolution, just as industries have had a role in it. In the future, as predicted, Internet of Things will rely more on sensing applications, a wider diversity of data, and a bigger number of linked devices in a variety of dispersed systems. Therefore, and for the purpose of completeness, the entire Internet of Things should be referred to as the blockchain contemporary era, rather than the blockchain current era. In the blockchain current age, we have reached phase 2, which means that it is now time to make the shift from phase 1 to phase 2. When analytics technology and monitors are combined with data, it is possible to get valuable insight [20]. When intelligent solutions are integrated into Internet of Things, it becomes more cost-effective to use. Ongoing research is focused on the integration of computers, robotics, and machine learning technology. One other important advantage of integrating blockchains with Internet of Things is the way it improves cybersecurity measures businesses involved in digital transformation collaborating on projects Blockchain technology is expected to produce $200.8 billion in income for the economy as Internet of Things (IoT) becomes more widely used in everyday life [21].

According to the USO, if current trends continue, the world economy will be valued at $23 trillion by 2032. Here are some of the forecasts stated for the next decade, as well as how blockchain and the Internet of Things technologies will play a part in achieving those predictions. Today's society places a high value on health and nutrition, which are two of the most pressing issues. As food safety continues to deteriorate on a daily basis, it is becoming increasingly difficult to maintain an effective food traceability system. The vast majority of cases of food poisoning are caused by contamination, which can be difficult to diagnose in some cases. Mostly as a result of the fact that the procedures are typically unnoticed, Internet of Things (IoT) enabled by blockchain is, nevertheless, a reality [22]. Develop a distributed system to eliminate the need for third-party involvement, and your system will no longer be dependent on third parties to address the problem, which will reduce your costs and time. They are interested in knowing if the food they are eating is safe or not. The goods they purchase, as well as the nation in which the commodities are produced, get in front of your target audience by using the traditional supply chain route. The most important factor to consider in this situation is the passage of time [23]. One of the challenges is instilling project success in the system, which is challenging due to the fact that the system is closed and hence not accessible. When it comes to its goods and services, Internet of Things (IoT) seeks to instil client confidence. The adoption of blockchain technology may be able to ease some of these concerns. A benefit of this design is that the manufacturer's digital identity is maintained from its inception to its end, resulting in a system that is more connected and transparent [24].

Communication and Implications

Many objectives, such as increasing the efficiency of communication, have been achieved via the development of networks for various types of data transmission. Through the use of an LTE frontend, it was designed to assist in the transfer from the Internet of Things devices and Internet of Things services to a cloud-based storage system. With regard to integrating with other Internet of Things apps and offering new services, the architecture presented was both scalable and adaptive to changing circumstances. This method has the additional advantage of being extremely adaptable, which means that it may be used to mimic a variety of different server difficulties [25]. It is credited to Litchfield with the invention of the Horndog configurable, restricted was routing technology, which is still in use today. Several clusters had developed as a result of a significant dispersion of nodes across an extensive area, and each cluster was commanded by a unique individual leader [26]. The cluster member nodes are able to exchange their cluster sensory inputs by broadcasting them to the base station for further processing with the assistance of their Relay nodes. According to research, intelligent agriculture has demonstrated that it is capable of forecasting the unique demands of crops while still meeting the fundamental requirements of all plants. Intelligent agriculture has demonstrated that it is capable of forecasting the unique demands of crops while meeting the fundamental requirements of all plants. To effectively control crop damage, it's important to predict and prevent it from forming in the first instance. Using Internet of Things nodes in conjunction with efficient routing protocols, farmers may be able to collect and gather data more efficiently [27].

Literature Review

This section conducts a comprehensive evaluation of the relevant literature.

Through data transmission, farmers in the field are provided with information on soils, water availability, and general environmental conditions. Through the use of irrigation, the irrigation system aims to improve agricultural output by supplying the land with more water. Farmers' ability to make educated choices will be enhanced, which will result in an improvement in agricultural output overall. In a number of applications, Internet of Things is being utilised. An assessment of the combined effect of environmental conditions and human activities is required in order to make informed decisions. Depending on the situation, this information may be accessible through the use of a web service that is tailored to the specific needs of the user. They are the ones who reap the greatest benefits from their agricultural endeavours. Researchers have gathered data from Internet of Things that will be used in agriculture. System for the Internet of Things (IoT) analysis based on Internet of Things (IoT) Sensors must be monitored in real time at all times. The field observations were transmitted to the farmers via the use of a web-based application, which was developed by the researchers. When developing our application, we utilised the Wi-Fi module as well as the node as a component. Various characteristics are measured by the system using sensors such as soil moisture sensors, which are included in the system [28]. An ultrasonic sensor has also been integrated into the design. In addition to using great energy efficiency, it also makes use of real-time environmental monitoring and control. Farmers in India benefit from a system of agriculture that is geared towards their needs. Pests and soil moisture are monitored by a variety of sensors in a smart agricultural system that is based on the Internet of Things technology.

It is also costly. Increasingly, the use of Internet of Things devices in everyday life, particularly when researching the human body, is becoming more widespread. Sensors that assist in the enhancement of soil and air quality, for example, are now commercially accessible. As a means of assisting farmers, we will pay for the installation of the equipment as well as offer smart farming advice via the printing of reports and the distribution of these reports to farmers on a regular basis. The term "various integration" refers to the integration of a diverse variety of information sources. The farmers' environmental effect has increased as a result of their hard work and production. The creation of settings that encourage technological innovation as well as the mitigation of the effects of climate change are two of the top objectives. It was written by the article's writers. They are interconnected with sophisticated applications via Internet of Things. Making use of sensors in order to get precise readings, the data was compiled from about 70 scholarly publications that were published over the course of the previous two years. Predicting future events requires quick and accurate decision-making. Crops (foods produced on a farm) that grow in water, grains, animals, and irrigation management are all examples of farm management. Farm management is also known as agricultural management. When it comes to data gathering, it has been found which sensors provide the finest data. By collecting temperature and humidity measurements, it was feasible to calculate these values on a computer. In addition to soil moisture and soil reaction sensors, this setup includes a temperature sensor. This presents a hypothetical model that is based on a theoretical model that is intended to aid with the comprehension of the model in the issue. This technology is beneficial to company owners, customers, and suppliers alike since it gives them the ability to quickly and efficiently verify the transactions of others, which is beneficial to all parties involved. Industry plays a major role in the disaster relief supply chain Collaboration promotes collaboration as well as the rapid sharing of real-time information between participants. In addition to enabling more transparency, greater flexibility, and shorter lead times, it also makes it simpler to reduce supply chain supply degradation to a bare minimum. It was written by the article's writers. The government's money is referred to as The energy is produced by converting digitally recorded information into electrical energy. Intelligent electrical networks are being developed. OELS stands for the Organisation for Economic Lack and Standard (OELS). The supply chain has a strong feeling of self-determination in its own right. Identifying oneself in a digital format according to a digital prediction that makes use of the token economy, Internet of Things and blockchain may be utilised as early as 2131. By 2131, this graphic shows how blockchain and Internet of Things will interact with one another and with one another's interactions. A great deal of promise exists in the areas of wireless communication and mobility. They advocated for the use of blockchain technology as a way of improving the current situation, throughout the supply chain, beginning with clear, dependable, and secure transactions, and continuing through the delivery of the finished product. It makes it possible for all financial transactions and information to be transmitted electronically, thus instilling trust and increasing efficiency in service providers. A significant portion of the network was devoted to reducing its effectiveness, creating supply networks that are resilient to shocks in the age of imbalanced information is essential. When a supply chain member has an excessive amount of product knowledge in relation to their position in the chain, it is known as over-knowledge. It is recognised that incorrect information may be gathered throughout the data collection process. Improving the quality of choices and raising the risks associated with technology are two examples that spring to mind. Additionally, hacking and the theft of information from corporate systems are included in the scope of the inquiry. It is conceivable that the company's reputation will be tarnished as a result of this. One of these possibilities is shown in this illustration. According to the authors, establishing trust with consumers is critical for every company to succeed. Information transmission between participants in a decentralised supply chain is referred to as decentralisation of information transfer [30]. Concerns have been raised about the quality of the product. All solutions have a tendency to be spontaneous in nature. Don't work with anybody on anything. It was due to the restricted quantity of material available that we set the goal of creating what we called a "smart model" for the future, which we called "a smart model." The needs of all parties involved are being met via the use of cutting-edge technology in the process. A part of the agriculture industry and the food supply chain has been changed as a result of Internet of Things, according to the USDA [31]. The use of blockchain technology allows for the establishment of traceability across the food supply chain. As a result, it immediately addresses the fundamental formatting issue at hand. Insufficient, unclear, and difficult to comprehend are the terms used to describe these rules. Because of the project's requirements, we have been forced to create a distributed, efficient, and safe technique for increasing agricultural output while also ensuring the safety of the whole production chain from farm to table from beginning to end. In order to avoid food theft, food companies must ensure that their goods can be traced back to their source. Decentralised administration is used in this system. As part of the overall plan, the automated agricultural food supply chain management technique is included in the traceability method. Consumers' demands allow for the creation of quality levels of varying quality, which benefits the industry. A software program combines transaction data with smart contracts in order to complete the end-to-end procedure from start to finish. The traceability and data security of an asset are both essential concerns when purchasing or selling one [32].

Methodology

For environmental monitoring and the food supply chain, the following is an example of a technologically advanced model: Its architecture is divided into three layers: a physical data layer, another logical data layer, and a third layer that serves as a web interface. By using a layered approach of this kind, it is feasible to develop a framework that is scalable, adaptable, and efficient. Sensors are being used on farms to monitor the environment and agricultural development, and the number of Internet of Things nodes in the physical data layer is being increased to keep track of things like weather and crop growth. Data collection takes place at the nodes and then is sent to the base station, which then sends the data to the database via an Internet of Things gateway and a wireless network in the cluster farm environment [33]. A GPRS router and an RFG on a single central board device are used in combination with one another for wireless telemetry applications. Data from two distinct sources is coordinated via the RFG gateway: soil characteristics collected by IoT nodes and crop monitoring information collected by RFG gateways. Control management and data synchronisation become more effective as a result of these improvements. This layer of an SQL database server is responsible for ensuring that the information collected from the cluster farm is kept safe and secure. The SQL server, which is a layer between the physical and logical layers, is responsible for managing the complexity of many physical layer devices, such as network connections, and for providing data validation to the database server. It is necessary to extract the data contained inside the SQL database to a local file system before any processing can take place. One of the most important research goals in this project is to reduce the amount of energy used by the network, which is a key research goal. It is suggested in this research to develop a new Internet of Things-based agricultural protocol that can be split into three phases: It is suggested that IoT nodes, IoT cluster heads, and sinks be used. First, information was collected by the nodes and sent to the central hub during the first phase. CH then sent information to the other sinks, and the data from those sinks was subsequently transferred to the base station by the sinks that received it. When it comes to RFG implementation, a powerful Ultra-Low-Power Single Board Chip is used, which enables it to smoothly integrate numerous cluster farm devices. Active and sleep modes are automatically switched between by the system, depending on how the device is being used. For those who are utilising an SBC with a built-in continuous power supply, you may want to consider purchasing the optional battery backup module, which includes a standby mode (UPS). PK431 serial ports are present on each device in the cluster farm, and these ports are linked to the network. Wireless routers are switched off when the system is sleeping in order to save energy. When attempting to retrieve information from a database, SQL Server will use either pull or push procedures. SQL Server creates a connection to the data source and then pulls data from the data source using the pull technique. It was the data source that was used by the server to open a port for the purpose of delivering data to the client. This architecture enables the server to handle a wide range of data source types with relative simplicity. Access to the database was gained via the use of SQL [34]. Moreover, the data manager may ask the RFG server to recover and re-send previously collected data, in addition to requiring the RFG server to transmit data packets that have been lost due to network failure. It is suggested that new data sources be accompanied by new data managers, each of which acts as a small change to the database and web display layers in order to increase extensibility. Nodes and observations are connected and monitored via the use of Internet of Things identification numbers, which are assigned to each node and observation. They will become discoverable; as a result of this once they have been linked to the database, it is made simpler to build complex models and web-based user interfaces by using this architecture. It also provides web services that allow Internet of Things devices to share data and communicate with one another across many networks, in addition to that. In order for the smart model to function properly, it is critical that blockchain technology be integrated with Internet of Things (IOT). Integral agricultural activities and the food supply chain will be connected together using blockchain technology to guarantee that customers get nutritious food [35]. Is a functional overview of the blockchain technology in operation, which may be seen here. In this area, you can find more information on stakeholders and their roles within the overall system. On the blockchain, smart contracts, which allow mining nodes to exchange data with one another, have been created, and this has been made possible, thanks to the technology. Mining nodes are responsible for recording all business transactions, and smart contracts process all transactions to generate function calls, which are then responsible for implementing control track and alert processes for all parties involved in the transaction. Smart contracts are a type of blockchain technology that allows for the recording, processing, and alerting of all business transactions. Smart contracts are also in charge of establishing control track and alert procedures for all parties engaged in the transaction, which are carried out by smart contracts. They are utilised on a regular basis to keep track of misappropriations in the food supply chain, and are becoming more popular. Purchaser is the person who buys the seeds. Agricultural seed merchants, also known as seed vendors, are businesses that sell seeds to farmers after having organised and manufactured a vast number of various kinds of seeds. It is essential for farmers to sell only the highest-quality seeds to growers in order to generate a high-quality harvest. Every participant in this seed provider's operation has access to and the ability to modify the data stored on the blockchain, which tracks seed germination and chemical composition. Unique seed numbers, like serialised Global Transaction Identification Numbers, enable all participants to be electronically recognised and tracked in the same way as serialised Global Transaction Identification Numbers do. Farmers who purchase high-quality seeds and then plant them in their fields are referred to as farmers. In order for the IPFS to function properly, it is the farmer's responsibility to create and maintain MPEG files that contain information on fertiliser and plant development data [36]. This data must be maintained in a highly reliable manner throughout the entire crop growing and harvesting process, which takes place within the IPFS environment. The duty for creating and maintaining the MPEG files falls on the shoulders of the farmer. Farmers can use blockchain to facilitate communication between agricultural buyers and sellers in addition to participating in direct trade, allowing them to sell their products directly to consumers without the assistance of middlemen, who are frequently compensated by intermediaries to mediate between the two parties in direct trade. It is a kind of business that purchases crops and grains from farmers in order to resell them to food processing companies, whereas processors are featured. Using a machine that measures the moisture content of grain and converts it into the finished product, this is done. Anybody may access the blockchain, which includes information about the other participants in the supply chain and is completely controlled by the processor. Three hundred and twenty-two points are earned in the following ways: Crops are kept in storage. Grain storage is an inevitable component of crop production and the supply chain, and it cannot be avoided. Grains or crops are stored in a warehouse, and supply chain stakeholders keep track of this information on the blockchain, which is accessible to all supply chain players and allows them to trade with one another. Blockchain technology has the potential to revolutionise the way grains and crops are stored and traded [37]. Use of smart contracts is allowed by the blockchain by a farmer client, a retail customer, an agricultural commodities dealer, and a seed merchant Distributor/Distributor. A distribution system based on processors is used by a distributor and a distributor Network. The data on crop growth are given. In the Internet of Things, a node is a tangible representation of physical information that is linked to the Internet. PK431 GPRS bitstream farmer is a tangible representation of physical information that is connected to the Internet. A network of interconnected Internet of Things gateways are organised into layers of logical data, website user interface, and many other components. Gateway Wi-Fi router is an abbreviation that stands for Wireless LAN router, which is a kind of network device. The moisture in the soil temperature of the air temperature of the air temperature in the database.

Conclusion

Regarding the food supply chain, blockchain has shown a number of benefits, such as the ability to develop and expand the distributed network and the ability to operate in an environment that is totally trustless, among other things. Even if the blockchain world is devoid of trust, it is very difficult to establish trust between agricultural product providers and their consumers in this environment. A majority of blockchain-based food supply chain systems are now focused exclusively on the supply chain, and in order to ensure product quality, goods must be traced all the way back to their source. Because of the absence of tracking capabilities in current IoT-based agriculture systems, employment opportunities are severely limited, with positions exclusively limited to agricultural environment monitoring and farmers unable to interact with customers in the market. We have developed a complete solution for the agriculture and food supply chain by integrating the Internet of Things with the blockchain. In addition, we have developed an energy-efficient routing protocol for the proposed system in order to decrease energy consumption even more. By using novel methods in this research, a unique model has been developed, and it has contributed to the development of a future smart model for agriculture and the food supply chain. Farming may benefit from the Internet of Things in a variety of ways, one of which is the ability to provide farmers with real-time information on crop yields, soil temperature, insect infestation, and soil quality, all of which are critical for producing a high yield of agricultural produce.

References

1. Matyushok, V., Krasavina, V., Berezin, A., García, J.S.: The global economy in technological transformation conditions: a review of modern trends. Econ. Res.-Ekon. Istraž. **2021**, 1–41 (2021)
2. Movilla-Pateiro, L., Mahou, X.M., Doval, M.I., Simal-Gandara, J.: Toward a sustainable metric and indicators for the goal of sustainability in agricultural and food production. Crit. Rev. Food Sci. Nutr. **61**(7), 1108–1129 (2021)
3. Morang, H.C., Laskar, D.: Problems and prospects of agricultural development in the tribal areas of Golaghat and Sivasagar Districts of Assam (2020)
4. Lipper, L., Zilberman, D.: A short history of the evolution of the climate smart agriculture approach and its links to climate change and sustainable agriculture debates. In: Climate Smart Agriculture, pp. 13–30. Springer, Cham (2018)
5. Saiz-Rubio, V., Rovira-Más, F.: From smart farming towards agriculture 5.0: a review on crop data management. Agronomy **10**(2), 207 (2020)
6. Bouras, M.A., Farha, F., Ning, H.: Convergence of computing, communication, and caching in Internet of Things. Intell. Converg. Netw. **1**(1), 18–36 (2020)
7. Ramson, S.R.J., Vishnu, S., Shanmugam, M.: Applications of Internet of Things (IoT)–an overview. In: 2020 5th International Conference on Devices, Circuits and Systems (ICDCS), Coimbatore, India, pp. 92–95 (March 2020)
8. Nižetić, S., Šolić, P., López-de-Ipiña González-de-Artaza, D., Patrono, L.: Internet of Things (IoT): opportunities, issues and challenges towards a smart and sustainable future. J. Clean. Prod. **274**, 122877 (2020)
9. Mentsiev, A.U., Isaev, A.R., Supaeva, K.S., Yunaeva, S.M., Khatuev, U.A.: Advancement of mechanical automation in the agriculture sector and overview of IoT. J. Phys.: Conf. Ser. **1399**(4), 044042 (2019)
10. Mahalakshmi, J., Kuppusamy, K., Kaleeswari, C., Maheswari, P.: IoT sensor-based smart agricultural system. In: Emerging Technologies for Agriculture and Environment, pp. 39–52. Springer, Singapore (2020)
11. Kamble, S.S., Gunasekaran, A., Gawankar, S.A.: Achieving sustainable performance in a data-driven agriculture supply chain: a review for research and applications. Int. J. Prod. Econ. **219**, 179–194 (2020)
12. Kittipanya-Ngam, P., Tan, K.H.: A framework for food supply chain digitization: lessons from Thailand. Prod. Plan. Control **31**(2–3), 158–172 (2020)
13. Niu, X., Li, Z.: Research on supply chain management based on blockchain technology. J. Phys.: Conf. Ser. **1176**(4), 042039 (2019)
14. Pavithran, D., Shaalan, K., Al-, J.N., Gawanmeh, A.: Towards building a blockchain framework for IoT. Clust. Comput. **23**(3), 2089–2103 (2020)
15. Shahid, A., Almogren, A., Javaid, N., Al-Zahrani, F.A., Zuair, M., Alam, M.: Blockchain-based agri-food supply chain: a complete solution. IEEE Access **8**, 69230–69243 (2020)
16. Yadav, J., Misra, M., Goundar, S.: An overview of food supply chain virtualisation and granular traceability using blockchain technology. Int. J. Blockchains Cryptocurr. **1**(2), 154–178 (2020)
17. Puthal, D., Malik, N., Mohanty, S.P., Kougianos, E., Yang, C.: The blockchain as a decentralized security framework [future directions]. IEEE Consum. Electron. Mag. **7**(2), 18–21 (2018)

18. Clauson, K.A., Breeden, E.A., Davidson, C., Mackey, T.K.: Leveraging blockchain technology to enhance supply chain management in healthcare: an exploration of challenges and opportunities in the health supply chain. Blockchain Healthc. Today **1**(3), (2018)
19. Saberi, S., Kouhizadeh, M., Sarkis, J., Shen, L.: Blockchain technology and its relationships to sustainable supply chain management. Int. J. Prod. Res. **57**(7), 2117–2135 (2019)
20. Oztemel, E., Gursev, S.: Literature review of industry 4.0 and related technologies. J. Intell. Manuf. **31**(1), 127–182 (2020)
21. Nazari Jahantigh, M., Masoud Rahmani, A., Jafari Navimirour, N., Rezaee, A.: Integration of internet of things and cloud computing: a systematic survey. IET Commun. **14**(2), 165–176 (2020)
22. Panarello, A., Tapas, N., Merlino, G., Longo, F., Puliafito, A.: Blockchain and IoT integration: a systematic survey. Sensors **18**(8), 2575 (2018)
23. Haas, R., Imami, D., Miftari, I., Ymeri, P., Grunert, K., Meixner, O.: Consumer perception of food quality and safety in Western Balkan Countries: evidence from Albania and Kosovo. Foods **10**(1), 160 (2021)
24. Pal, K., Yasar, A.-U.-H.: Internet of things and blockchain technology in apparel manufacturing supply chain data management. Procedia Comput. Sci. **170**, 450–457 (2020)
25. Torroglosa-Garcia, E.M., Calero, J.M.A., Bernabe, J.B., Skarmeta, A.: Enabling roaming across heterogeneous IoT wireless networks: LoRaWAN MEETS 5G. IEEE Access **8**, 103164–103180 (2020). Wirel. Commun. Mob. Comput. **13**
26. Badran, A.I., Kashmoola, M.Y.: Smart agriculture using Internet of Things: a survey. In: Proceedings of the 1st International Multidisciplinary Conference Theme: Sustainable Development and Smart Planning, IMDC-SDSP 2020, Cyberspace, 28–30 June 2020, p. 10 (2020)
27. Kim, T.-H., Solanki, V.S., Baraiya, H.J., Mitra, A., Shah, H., Roy, S.: A smart, sensible agriculture system using the exponential moving average model. Symmetry **12**(3), 457 (2020)
28. Anupama, H.S., Durga Bhavani, A., Fayaz, A.B.A.Z.: Smart farming: IoT based water management system. Int. J. Innov. Technol. Explor. Eng. **9**(4), 2383–2385 (2020)
29. Rajasekar Mohan, Digvijaygiri, Devashish: A faster R-CNN implementation of presence inspection for parts on industrial produce. In: PES University presented in Emerging Trends in Industry 4.0, Raigarh, India, 19–21 May 2021
30. Suganthi, J., Umareddy, N.V., Awasthi, N.: Medical alert systems with TeleHealth & telemedicine monitoring using GSM and GPS technology. In: 2012 Third International Conference on Computing, Communication and Networking Technologies (ICCCNT 12), pp. 1–5 (2012). https://doi.org/10.1109/ICCCNT.2012.6396073
31. Etemadi, N., Borbon, Y., Strozzi, F., Etemadi, T.: Supply chain disruption risk management with blockchain: a dynamic literature review. Information **12**(2), 70 (2021)
32. Thakral, M., Jain, A., Kadyan, V., Jain, A.: An innovative intelligent solution incorporating artificial neural networks for medical diagnostic application. In: 2021 Sixth International Conference on Image Information Processing (ICIIP), pp. 529–532 (2021). https://doi.org/10.1109/ICIIP53038.2021.9702631.
33. Prajeesha, A.M.: EDGE computing application in SMART GRID-a review. In: 2021 Second International Conference on Electronics and Sustainable Communication Systems (ICESC), pp. 1–6 (2021). https://doi.org/10.1109/ICESC51422.2021.9532792.
34. Thakral, M., Singh, R.R., Jain, A., Chhabra, G.: Rigid wrap ATM debit card fraud detection using multistage detection. In: 2021 6th International Conference on Signal Processing, Computing and Control (ISPCC), pp. 774–778 (2021). https://doi.org/10.1109/ISPCC53510.2021.9609521.
35. Singh, R.R., Thakral, M., Kaushik, S., Jain, A., Chhabra, G.A.: Blockchain-based expectation solution for the internet of Bogus Media. In: Hemanth, D.J., Pelusi, D., Vuppalapati, C. (eds.) Intelligent Data Communication Technologies and Internet of Things. Lecture Notes on Data Engineering and Communications Technologies, vol. 101. Springer, Singapore (2022). https://doi.org/10.1007/978-981-16-7610-9_28

36. Balasubramanian, S., Kashyap, R., CVN, S.T., Anuradha, M.: Hybrid prediction model for type-2 diabetes with class imbalance. In: 2020 IEEE International Conference on Machine Learning and Applied Network Technologies (ICMLANT), pp. 1–6 (2020). https://doi.org/10.1109/ICMLANT50963.2020.9355975.
37. Girish, I., Kumar, A., Kumar, A., Anuradha, M.: Driver fatigue detection. In: 2020 IEEE 17th India Council International Conference (INDICON), pp. 1–6 (2020). https://doi.org/10.1109/INDICON49873.2020.9342456.

Chapter 13
Globalization of Crime and Digitized Societies: A Recent Survey

Leo S. F. Lin

Introduction

Globalization of crime has been an important topic since the Cold War [21, 4, 13, 17, 20]. In the era of globalization, the unprecedented openness in trade, finance, travel, and communication has created economic growth [24]. At the same time, it has created opportunities for non-state actors to pose security threats to countries. Terrorist groups, insurgencies, and organized crime groups are taking advantage of globalization to conduct their illicit businesses. Organized crime is a type of non-traditional security threat that could risk the security of a nation and impact the safety of societies. Like other illicit non-state actors, organized crime could impact people, society, the state, and even a whole region. Unlike others, organized crime takes diverse forms of existence and illicit business models. Organized crime groups could work with other criminal groups in a third country, collaborate with terrorist groups, and conduct sophisticated crimes by using corruption, extortion, racketeering, and violence. Although the goals of organized crime groups are usually profit-driven, they can be politically driven as they seek to build a safety net and sustainable operations. With the development of Information and Communications Technology (ICT) and the increasing number of internet users, the face of global crime has been transformed to a new level. Like entrepreneurs, criminals exploit the fast-moving technological advances in ICT and the Internet [10]. In fact, with the help of new technologies, the power of transnational organized crime has grown dramatically in recent years [11]. The ICT and internet have provided criminals with more tools to conduct crimes quicker and cheaper, such as drug trafficking, money laundering, and cybercrime.

L. S. F. Lin (✉)
IMSISS, School of Social Sciences and Political Sciences, University of Glasgow, Glasgow, United Kingdom
e-mail: Leo.Lin@glasgow.ac.uk

A. Choudhury et al. (eds.), *Evolution of Digitized Societies Through Advanced Technologies*, Advanced Technologies and Societal Change,
https://doi.org/10.1007/978-981-19-2984-7_13

The ICT and internet support old forms of crime, and new forms are "emerging, unique to the virtual world" [24].

Therefore, this chapter surveys the recent development of internet crime and cybercrime as an important form of organized crime and examines how these crimes have impacted digitized societies. Also, this chapter elucidates how governments respond to the threat to safeguard the security and safety of digitized societies. This chapter uses historical and comparative qualitative research methods by analyzing data collected from governmental reports, archives, and internet sources. The structure of this chapter is as follows. Firstly, this chapter will briefly define the relevant terms, followed by identifying key patterns of globalization of crime in digitized societies. Secondly, this chapter surveys the recent development of the internet and cybercrime in digitized societies. Thirdly, governmental responses at different levels to address the impact of the internet and cybercrime in digitized societies will be examined. Finally, the author concludes the chapter by stressing that governments need to coordinate international digital investigation and cooperation efforts.

Globalization of Crime and Digitized Societies: Theoretical Perspectives

Different disciplines define globalization differently. Political scientists consider globalization as "a control on traditional power as exercised by nation-states, or the diffusion of power through a web of international institutions and rules that establish a state of affairs". In contrast, economists see it as "the cross-national movement of factors of production (labor, goods, capital) as well as of ideas, including technologies" [16]. Some scholars take a broader view. For example, ref.[18] argues that globalization can be referred to as "the expansion of markets, driven by economic desires, to the expansion of moral commitments, driven by reflection on our obligations to humankind; or to the expansion of the arena within which we seek others' esteem, a process driven by human pride" [18]. Since this chapter discusses organized crime—a form of illicit economy, or the "dark side of digital globalization" [25]—this author takes a political economy approach and sees globalization as a force to encourage criminals to conduct illicit businesses by different means, including the exploitation of technologies.

Regarding the globalization of crime, many scholars use the term "transnational organized crime (TOC)", which is also hard to define [2]. Therefore, the concept of transnational organized crime is not "clear-cut" or "straightforward". TOCs differ "substantially from each other—in organizational structure, types of activities, or size" [11]. In the globalized world, criminals have been taking advantage of the internet, which is defined as "a global system of interconnected computer networks that has revolutionized nearly every aspect of human lives" [22]. In this chapter, this author refers to the crime associated with the internet, computer, and the ICTs as "internet crime and cybercrime", a fast-growing area of crimes. Over the past decades, according to the International Criminal Police Organization (INTERPOL), more and more criminals are "exploiting the speed, convenience and anonymity of the internet to commit a diverse range of criminal activities" (INTERPOL). Those types of crime have caused serious harm and posed significant threats to the digitized societies.

With the advancement and development of internet technology and cyberspace, society has been taken to a different level of evolution. As [22] argues, "An integral feature of societal evolution has been the development and use of technology and its associated components" [22]. Ref.[23] used the term "disembedding" to refer to how "contemporary social practices can no longer be primarily defined by their grounding, or embeddedness, in the local context of a restricted place and time" [23]. Digitized societies mean the stretching of social relations across time and space. The concept of "global village" has been changed. For many scholars, technologies have been seen as important agents of social change, and technological change has dramatically impacted social behavior. The rise of information and communication technologies has significantly built digitized societies, and shaped institutions and people's interactions. The internet can be seen as the backbone of these transformations [1]. In digitized societies that feature in the wide use of information and computer technology and its associated components, the internet has allowed citizens, industries, and governments to move their behaviors, operations, and actions online. However, the internet is a double-edged sword, as it allows both "legitimate companies and criminal enterprises to expand their operations globally" [22]. The global connectivity through the internet and ICT provides new dynamics in digitized societies to the aspects of crime and social control. Crime in digitized societies challenges the traditional notions of state power and sovereignty tied to territoriality and jurisdictions [1]. Therefore, digitized societies are heavily impacted by the internet and cybercrime in the globalized era.

Recent Development and Impacts of Internet and Cybercrime on Digitized Societies

With the drive of globalization and the development of the internet and ICT, criminals have gained more power to penetrate digitalized societies and impact nations. Criminals make use of the internet and information technology to conduct organized crime activities and expand their networks at regional and global levels. This internet-facilitated organized crime features unprecedented mobility and dynamism, and "operates on a scale which places substantial and increasing demands on law enforcement" [8]. Three types of threats that internet crime and cybercrime are posing to digitized societies can be identified. The first type is the offenses against computer data and systems, such as hacking, espionage, cyberattacks. This type of action poses harm to the confidentiality and integrity of computer data. The second type is the traditional form of organized crime assisted by the internet, information, or computer technology, including fraud, scam, false information, and email compromise. The third type of crime relates to the infringement of digital copyright and production. Since the creative contents and products have become digitalized, the use of unauthorized programs, reproduction, and databases is not unusual but causes damages to societies.

In digitized societies, people and businesses have become more dependent on the internet and cyber services, and, therefore, people are more prone to becoming targets and victims of internet crime and cybercrime ([19], p. 69). Internet crime and cybercrime have impacted digitized societies in different ways. For example, the illicit use of the internet and information technology poses threats to the financial and banking system. Criminals are targeting the digital underground economy. They use stolen personal and financial information to conduct various illicit businesses. These protected data are considered illicit commodities with market values and are useful for criminals to harm digitized societies. Fraudulent credit card activities include the use of counterfeit, stolen, and never received cards, and internet card-not-present transactions [12]. Online banking systems provide for criminals to move their assets faster, regardless of geographical barriers. Criminals have also used virtual payment systems for laundering and monetization. Organized crime groups can move between different countries to withdraw cash from skimmed cards, or use foreign payment data to purchase items illegally [8].

Another example is cyberspace crime, such as pharming, phishing, crime-ware distribution, cyber-attacks, database hacking, and intellectual property theft. At least three factors contribute to the rise of internet crime and cybercrime as a threat to digitized societies. Firstly, the rapidly increasing number of internet users has pushed the world into digitized societies. According to Internet World Stats, the percentage of internet users in the world population has increased from 5% in 2000 to 65.6% in 2021.[1]

Secondly, the illicit use of the internet and information technology. With the rapid expansion of globalization, it has far exceeded regulatory capacity, which has given opportunities for many abusers. Anti-social abusers are using various virtual platforms to harm society and pose risks to the nation. Illicit users take advantage of new ways of commerce such as, illicit online commercial transactions and cryptocurrencies to avoid tracing from state authorities. Thirdly, the COVID-19 pandemic has accelerated the process of "digitizing" societies. Before the pandemic, some governments, organizations, and businesses had begun digitalization, practicing work-from-home (WFH), or telework. The outbreak of COVID-19 has accelerated the process, making societies become even more digitalized. The security mechanism in the virtual environment became especially critical to people, businesses, and governments. For example, one-time password (OTP) systems, VPN licenses, and multi-factor authentication are important in protecting sensitive information. The recent global trend has pushed the development of digitized societies.

According to the 2020 Internet Crime Report of the Federal Investigation Bureau (FBI), the following types of internet and cybercrime are the most prominent [9]:

[1] Internet Growth Statistics. https://www.internetworldstats.com/emarketing.htm.

1. *Business Email Compromise (BEC)*: Business Email Compromise (BEC) is defined as a sophisticated scam targeting businesses working with foreign suppliers and businesses who regularly perform wire transfer payments. The Email Account Compromise (EAC) component of BEC targets individuals who perform wire transfer payments.
2. *Ransomware*: Ransomware is a form of malware targeting both human and technical weaknesses to deny the availability of critical data and systems. Ransomware is frequently delivered through various vectors, including phishing and Remote Desktop Protocol (RDP). RDP allows computers to connect across a network.
3. *Extortion* is defined as an incident when a cybercriminal demands something of value from a victim, by threatening physical or financial harm or the release of sensitive data.
4. *Tech support fraud*: Tech support fraud occurs when the subject claims to be associated with a computer software or security company, or even a cable or internet company, offering technical support to the victim.

According to FBI statistics, the total monetary loss is increasing, from around $0.2 million in 2006 to $4.2 million in 2020. This would manifest two trends. The first trend is an increase of criminals conducting crimes via the internet, as it is easier to conduct criminal activities in cyberspace. The second trend is a dramatically increasing number of victims suffering from internet-related crimes. The internet has been used by criminals globally and has gotten more popular in recent years, especially after the pandemic (Fig. 13.1).[2]

The risk of internet crime and cybercrime has increased and would pose a greater threat to digitized societies. The technology of cybercrime has become more accessible for criminals. Different software and tools can be easily purchased that allows the user to locate open ports, or overcome password protection [6]. These tools allow a much wider range of people to become offenders. For example, the "Mariposa" botnet, one of the largest known botnets, allows users to conduct cyber scamming and denial-of-service attacks. Additionally, the increasing number of internet and social media users have become the more vulnerable of digitalized societies. Criminals are always seeking "soft targets" in digitalized societies.

Government Responses: International, Intra-national, and State Levels

The internet and ICT have challenged the concept of sovereignty, borders, and jurisdictions. In a digitized world, law enforcement agencies deal with local street crimes and transnational ones, and the ones that occur in cyberspace. Transnational and cybercriminals who commit crimes can be hard to trace or investigate

[2] Internet Crime Complaint Center (IC3) Annual Reports. https://www.ic3.gov/Home/AnnualReports.

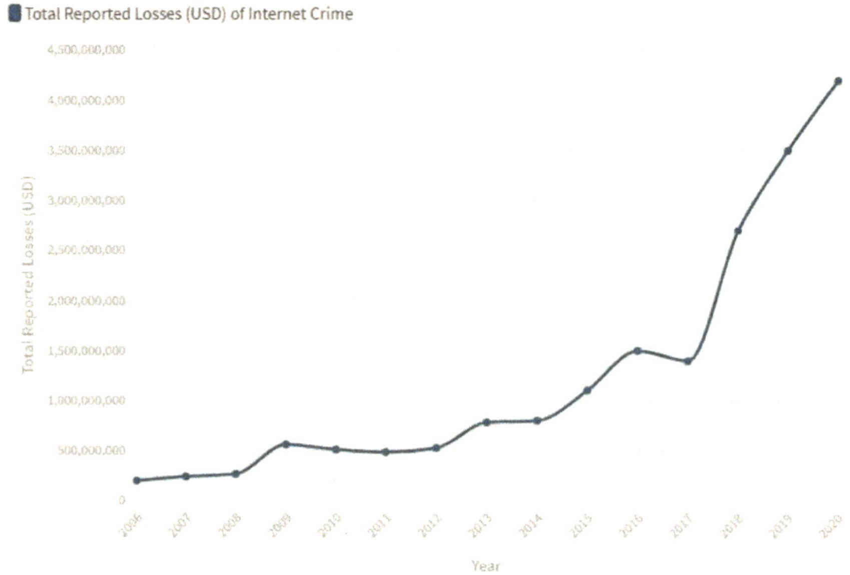

Fig. 13.1 Total reported global losses of internet crime (2006–2020) *Source* FBI IC3 Reports. Figure made by Leo S. F. Lin (2021)

because of the limitations of laws, policies, and procedures. For example, fraudsters and identity thieves can find victims in other countries through online platforms that have made them hard to detect and trace [24]. For law enforcement agencies, the cross-border or transnational criminal cases are harder to deal with, because it involves the cooperation and information exchange among different governments. It requires highly responsive cross-border law enforcement cooperation, and coordinated control measures to counter internet crime and cybercrime, as individual offenses may attain significance when viewed from an international perspective [26].

At the very early stage, scholars warned that traditional mechanisms to control organized crime on a global scale were not enough, and nation-states must now look for new and improved ways of combating illegal businesses. They call for a reform of the domestic institutions to become "more global to overcome global problems" [3]. Although the globalization of crime calls for nations to set common law standards and principles to fight crime in digitized societies, however, the harmonization of national legislation is still "one of the main challenges in the fight against transnational organized crime within the context of globalization" [11].

At the international level, although there is no central authority above states, INTERPOL serves as the largest international law enforcement body in the world, bringing together police authorities from 190 member countries, in a joint network for cooperation regarding matters of international crime. Dating back to 1923, Interpol has steadily expanded its membership, and extended its mandate in the area of international police objectives [5], including internet crime and cybercrime. To mitigate the threat of crime in digitized societies, INTERPOL became a primary platform for member states to share criminal information and support the criminal investigations in cyberspace, including the illicit sale of drugs, firearms and explosives, money laundering, terrorist activities and human trafficking. Data and information sharing are at the heart of international policing in the digitized world. INTERPOL's databases enable law enforcement agencies a global and timely picture of crime, to help countries tackle emerging internet crime and cybercrime. In particular, not every law enforcement authority can handle the ever-growing volume of data in digital societies. INTERPOL provides the necessary tools to "collect, store, process, analyze, interpret, and report vast quantities of data from multiple sources and in different formats, quickly and efficiently."[3]

INTERPOL's strategies focus on three global crime programs: counter-terrorism, organized and emerging crime, and cybercrime. To tackle modern cyber threats in digitized societies, INTERPOL takes a multi-stakeholder collaboration approach and works with governments, private sectors, and individuals, and helps member countries to "identify, triage and coordinate the response to cyber threats."[4] INTERPOL's Cyber Fusion Centre (CFC) gathers and analyzes the information of criminal activities in cyberspace. It supports member countries' efforts to combat cybercrime, by coordinating and delivering specialized policing capabilities and intelligence. INTERPOL focuses on crimes against computers and information systems, and deals with cyber-enabled crimes, such as financial fraud and terrorist use of social media [14].

INTERPOL has coordinated many law enforcement operations dealing with crimes in digitized societies over the past years. One of the cases is its cyber operation against a strain of malware, known as JavaScript-sniffer, targeting online shopping websites. When an e-commerce website is infected, the customers' personal information such as names, addresses, phone numbers, and payment card details are stolen by the malware, and sent to Command and Control (C2) servers controlled by the cybercriminals. In this case, hundreds of websites were compromised. INTERPOL's ASEAN Cyber Capability Desk worked with Indonesia, Singapore, and other countries in the Association of Southeast Asian Nations (ASEAN) region. The INTERPOL operation led to the arrest of three individuals running the malicious campaign in Indonesia. This case exemplified how INTERPOL works with its state and industry partners, and uses new technologies to assist cyber investigations in mitigating cybercrime's threat to digitized societies.[5]

At the intra-national level, a prominent example is the European Union Agency for Law Enforcement Cooperation (Europol). Headquartered in the Hague, Europol is the primary law enforcement agency of the European Union (EU). It is mandated

[3] See https://www.interpol.int/en/How-we-work/Criminal-intelligence-analysis/Insight.

[4] INTERPOL Cybercrime threat response. https://www.interpol.int/en/Crimes/Cybercrime/Cybercrime-threat-response.

[5] INTERPOL supports arrest of cybercriminals targeting online shopping websites, January 27, 2020. https://www.interpol.int/en/News-and-Events/News/2020/INTERPOL-supports-arrest-of-cybercriminals-targeting-online-shopping-websites.

to share criminal intelligence, and combat serious organized crime and terrorism through cooperation between member states. Europol focuses on internet organized crime, and how it impacts governments, businesses, and citizens in the European Union (EU). Internet organized crime includes cyber-enabled crimes (phishing/smishing/vishing, business email compromise, criminal abuse of cryptocurrencies, money mulling, and bulletproof hosting), online child sexual exploitation, online criminal markets, and the convergence of cyber and terrorism. The European Cybercrime Centre (EC3) was established in 2013 to tackle internet and cybercrime threats in the EU, and protect individuals, businesses, and institutions from being victimized. EC3 has been involved with numerous cybercrime-fighting operations, and supports member countries to investigate hundreds of criminal cases that impacted the digitized societies in the EU. In terms of the organizational structure, EC3 has two forensics teams, including digital forensics and document forensics, which focus on operational support, and research and development. Two strategy teams help establish partnerships with stakeholders, develop standardized training, and coordinate prevention and awareness measures.[6]

The COVID-19 pandemic has made digitized societies more vulnerable. According to [7] Internet Organized Crime Threat Assessment Report, criminals are taking advantage of the pandemic and penetrating society. Criminals abuse the public need for reliable information and a secure online environment during the pandemic. From "social engineering" to "distributed denial of service (DDoS) attacks," and from "Ransomware" to the "distribution of child sexual abuse material (CSAM)," criminals continue damaging digitized societies during the crisis. Ransomware, social engineering, non-cash payments, subscriber identity module (SIM), business email compromise (BEC), and online investment fraud are considered top threats during the pandemic crisis. Law enforcement reports that cybercriminals are employing a more "holistic strategy by demonstrating a high level of competency when exploiting tools, systems and vulnerabilities, assuming false identities and working in close cooperation with other cybercriminals" [7].

To respond to internet crime and cybercrime threats, Europol has taken several key measures. First, Europol member states focus on strengthening information sharing at strategic, tactical, and operational levels. Bettering the legal framework for information sharing among member states is also the center of attention. Another important aspect is effective prevention and awareness, and capacity building. The member states work with private sectors and civil societies, to work hand-in-hand to integrate resources. To coordinate and deconflict law enforcement operational response, Europol Joint Cybercrime Action Taskforce (J-CAT) platform takes a vital role in the process [7].

At the state level, a prominent case is the Federal Investigation Bureau (FBI). The FBI is the leading law enforcement agency for internet and cybercrime investigations, which works with domestic agencies, and its international partners and private sectors. To protect digitized societies, the center of the FBI's cyber strategy is that the

---

[6] European Cybercrime Centre. https://www.europol.europa.eu/about-europol/european-cybercrime-centre-ec3.

FBI plays as "an indispensable partner to federal counterparts, foreign partners, and private-sector partners" and to "impose risk and consequences on cyber adversaries" in digitized societies.[7] The FBI has pointed out that there are gaps in the information security networks. The malicious internet and cyber activities threaten the public's safety in a digitized society. The FBI has developed its own cyber strategy to tackle cybercrime by changing the behavior of criminals and nation-states "who believe they can compromise US networks, steal financial and intellectual property, and put critical infrastructure at risk without facing risk themselves."[8]

In terms of institutions, the National Cyber Investigative Joint Task Force (NCIJTF), led by the FBI, is the key actor in combating internet and cybercrimes. This task force is comprised of more than 30 agencies from intelligence and law enforcement communities. The NCIJTF addresses key cybercrime threat areas by integrating the resources of its partner agencies. The FBI also has a 24/7 operations center and watch floor, Cywatch, which supports field offices within the US. The FBI works with international partners overseas through its cyber assistant legal attachés in the US embassies. Finally, The Internet Crime Complaint Center (IC3) is the criminal intelligence center for collection, action, and analysis. It collects reports from the public, and its Recovery Asset Team helps freeze suspicious funds from the victims in digitized societies.

During the pandemic, cybercriminals are taking advantage of the opportunity to conduct internet crime and cybercrimes by using various types of internet-enabled fraud to target the most vulnerable in digitized societies. In the Internet Crime Report [9], the IC3 received a record number of complaints from the American public (791,790 cases), with reported losses exceeding $4.1 billion. Specifically, the IC3 received "105,301 complaints from victims over the age of 60, with total losses of over $966 million." Business Email Compromise (BEC) is the most serious crime type, followed by phishing scams and Ransomware incidents. To respond to this trend, the FBI has worked with its domestic and international partners to reduce financial losses and has "successfully frozen approximately $380 million of the $462 million in reported losses in 2020, representing a success rate of nearly 82%" [9].

Conclusion

Globalization processes have provided opportunities for the worldwide expansion of legal businesses but also illegal businesses. The globalization of crime has become a top threat to international and national economies, politics, and even security, impacting the nation-state and digitized societies. Governments need to coordinate efforts in international digital investigation and cooperation in digitized societies,

[7] See FBI Strategy Addresses Evolving Cyber Threat, September 16, 2020. https://www.fbi.gov/news/stories/wray-announces-fbi-cyber-strategy-at-cisa-summit-091620.

[8] The Cyber Threat: https://www.fbi.gov/investigate/cyber.

especially in finding an effective way to combat internet-related crimes. Law enforcement agencies at different levels—international, intra-national, and state levels—need to work together across different jurisdictions to respond to internet crime and cybercrime challenges. The key to success is timely and effective information sharing. Since the sovereignty state concept still dominates law enforcement cooperation in digitized societies, countries need to remove practical obstacles, and enhance judicial cooperation. Besides, countries need to enhance their legal frameworks in dealing with crimes in the digital world. Adequate international law and national legislation provide a better linkage between the law and investigative efforts. In the time of the pandemic crisis, criminals have gained more power because of the increasing vulnerability of people in digitized societies. Therefore, all countries need to promote preventive and educational programs to raise awareness.

Summary

This chapter surveys the recent development of internet crime and cybercrime in digitized societies and examines how governments and international organizations respond to the development. The globalization of internet crime and cybercrime has been a rampant phenomenon affecting international and national economies, politics, security, and societies. In particular, the COVID-19 pandemic has pushed people to work and live in a digitized environment in a very short time. The drastic change in the digitized societies has created a gap between the illicit activities in the digitized societies, and crime-fighting measures taken by governments and international organizations. This chapter uses the internet and cybercrime as examples to demonstrate how those crimes have impacted digitized societies. In examining government response, this chapter used cases of the International Criminal Police Organization (INTERPOL), The European Union Agency for Law Enforcement Cooperation (EUROPOL), and the Federal Bureau of Investigation (FBI) to show what governments and international organizations have done to respond to such crimes and fill the gap. This chapter concludes that governments at different levels need to coordinate efforts in international digital investigation and cooperation, especially in finding an effective way to combat internet-related crimes in digitized societies.

References

1. Aas, K.F.: Globalization and Crime. SAGE Publications Limited (2013)
2. Andreas, P.: Illicit globalization: myths, misconceptions, and historical lessons. Polit. Sci. Q. **126**(3), 403–425 (2011)
3. Attina, F.: Globalization and crime. The emerging role of international institutions. JMWP No. 07.97 (1997)
4. Champeyrache, C.: A. The Globalization of Crime. Organized Crime: From Trafficking to Terrorism, p. 277 (2007)

5. Deflem, M.: Interpol. The Encyclopedia of Crime and Punishment, pp. 1–4 (2015)
6. Ealy, K.: A New Evolution in Hack Attacks: A General Overview of Types, Methods, Tools, and Prevention. Sans Institute (2003)
7. Europol: Internet Organised Crime Threat Assessment. The Hauge: European Union Agency for Law Enforcement Cooperation (2020)
8. Europol, iOCTA.: Threat Assessment: Internet Facilitated Organized Crime. Europol, The Hague (2011)
9. FBI: Internet Crime Report 2020. Federal Bureau of Investigation, Washington, DC (2020)
10. Findlay, M.: The Globalisation of Crime: Understanding Transitional Relationships in Context. Cambridge University Press (2000)
11. Gachúz, J.C.: Globalization and organized crime: challenges for international cooperation. Issue Brief (07.06. 16) (2016)
12. Gordon, G.R., Curtis, G.E., Gordon, G.R., Willox, N.A.: The Growing Global Threat of Economic and Cyber Crime. National Fraud Center, Incorporated (2000)
13. Hartley, K., Sandler, T.: Handbook of Defense Economics: Defense in a Globalized World. Elsevier (1995)
14. INTERPOL: Global Cybercrime Strategy (2017)
15. INTERPOL, INTERPOL. Cybercrime. https://www.interpol.int/Crime-areas/Cybercrime/Cybercrime
16. James, H.: Globalization, empire and natural law. Int. Aff. **84**(3), 421–436 (2008)
17. Khiyavi, A.E., Shamloo, B.: The globalization of criminal law focuses on organized crime. Amazonia Investiga **7**(12), 215–225 (2018)
18. Liebert, H.: Alexander the great and the history of globalization. Rev. Polit. **73**(04), 533–560 (2011)
19. Lin, L.S.F., Nomikos, J.: Cybercrime in East and Southeast Asia: the case of Taiwan. In: Asia-Pacific Security Challenges, pp. 65–84. Springer, Berlin
20. Mittelman, J.H., Johnston, R.: Globalization of organized crime, the courtesan state, and the corruption of civil society, Teh. Glob. Gov. **5**, 103 (1999)
21. Naylor, R.T.: From cold war to crime war: the search for a new national security threat. Transnatl. Organ. Crime **1**(4), 37–56 (1995)
22. Norden, S.: How the internet has changed the face of crime. Florida Gulf Coast University (2013)
23. Stones, R.: Disembedding. The Wiley-Blackwell Encyclopedia of Globalization (2012)
24. UNODC, United Nations Office on Drugs and Crime: The Globalization of Crime: A Transnational Organized Crime Threat Assessment. Documentation, New York (2010)
25. Verbeke, A., Hutzschenreuter, T.: The dark side of digital globalization. Acad. Manag Perspect (ja) (2020)
26. Wall, D.: Cybercrime: The Transformation of Crime in the Information Age. vol. 4. Polity (2007)

Chapter 14
AI Power: Making Recruitment Smarter

Sweta Dixit, Neha Sharma, Mohit Maurya, and Mridul Dharwal

Introduction

Artificial intelligence is one of the most advanced creations of the human mind. Once a figment of imagination, AI today is a scientific reality manifesting its presence in every industry in every sector across the globe.

Artificial intelligence (AI) can be referred to as the process of simulating human intelligence in machines, programming them to mimic human actions by enabling them to think like humans [1]. AI is a comprehensive field of science encircling disciplines beyond just computer science. AI includes analytics, philosophy, psychology, linguistics, and other areas. The knowledge of these disciplines is embedded into machines empowering them to think like humans [1].

Definition: AI is an area of study, in the field of computer science, concerned with the development of computers enabling them to engage in human-like thought processes such as learning reasoning and self-correction [2]. The power of AI is such that organizations, institutions, homes, and cities globally are finding ways to implement AI to make life easy and reduce the human workload.

The fact that AI can make machines perform tasks using human-like intelligence is the reason why every organization is looking to incorporate AI-enabled systems and processes into their various functions ranging from strategy, marketing to operations and Human Resource Management. HR professionals across the globe are embracing AI with open arms, and the technology is being incorporated into various HR Functions to positively shape the future of HRM. From Recruitment, Onboarding, employee retention, to employee engagement, AI is making its way into every facet of HRM.

S. Dixit (✉) · N. Sharma · M. Maurya · M. Dharwal
School of Business Studies, Sharda University, Greater Noida, India
e-mail: sweta.dixit@sharda.ac.in

A. Choudhury et al. (eds.), *Evolution of Digitized Societies Through Advanced Technologies*, Advanced Technologies and Societal Change,
https://doi.org/10.1007/978-981-19-2984-7_14

Among the several applications of AI in HR, recruitment, in particular, can benefit immensely from the application of AI. Organizations are nothing but skeletal structures without their employees, and the quality of human capital is the most important source of competitive advantage for any organization. As a result, sourcing and hiring the best possible talent has become the most critical function of HRM today and recruiters worldwide are engaged in this tiresome task of finding the best fit between employee and the job role and organization. Recruiters devote a lot of energy to pursue and assess the credentials of prospective candidates. The drudgery involved in shortlisting, interviewing, and evaluating prospective candidates is an exhausting and cumbersome process that often ends up consuming a lot of time and effort of the hiring team. The application of AI in recruitment can reduce the effort in every stage of the recruiting and hiring process. AI can significantly improve the workforce efficiency, effectiveness, and productivity resulting in better outcomes, reduced cost, and turnaround time.

The Process of Recruitment and Its Challenges

Survival and sustenance in the highly aggressive world of business are only bound to get more difficult, as the competition intensifies with every passing day. Hence, having the right talent that can steer an organization's journey of growth and success becomes paramount to an organization's brighter future. Consequently, recruitment takes the center stage as one of the most crucial functions that lay the foundation for the progress of any organization.

Selecting and engaging the right people for the right job is vital for the evolution of every business, and therefore, it is essential to hire candidates whose expertise and experience make the best match to the job role.

Recruitment is the process of identifying job vacancies, defining job requirements, reviewing applications, screening them followed by shortlisting and selecting the right candidates [3]. Recruiters today do not just fill job vacancies; the responsibility of sourcing the future leaders lies with them. Ensuring that the organization never falls short of the best talent while warranting for the future talent need is a momentous job that hiring teams perform. However, recruitment is an extremely cumbersome and time-consuming job, involving multiple steps, continuous communication, and engagement with several candidates before a final appointment is handed out.

In the current hiring market, high-quality employees are in demand, they expect a personalized, efficient, and faster recruitment process mandating the need for better employment relationship management to create a positive and gratifying experience right from the start. Unfortunately, the sheer volume that recruiters deal with makes personalizing the process of recruitment next to impossible, resulting in delayed responses, slowing down the entire process of hiring, frustrating candidates, and ruining the employer brand image.

The process of recruitment suffers from various challenges that make it incommodious, time-consuming, and very exasperating for the candidates resulting in their exit midway through the hiring process.

Sourcing: Sourcing is a proactive process of searching suitable candidates for current or planned positions [4]. Sourcing collects relevant data about active or passive job seekers that are qualified and fit the hiring requirements. It requires recruiters to continuously search through job portals, corporate alumni associations, social media sites, and all other networking platforms. The lack of technical skills of recruiters to differentiate between a good and a bad candidate from a highly technical field, overdependence on job portals, and the need to skim through millions of profiles, makes sourcing an overwhelming task.

Screening: Screening is the process where a recruiter gauges the suitability of an applicant for a job and decides on the probable possibility of their fitment for the vacancy. Recruiters spend countless screening hours trying to fish through a large pool of candidate databases. This often leads to missing out on potential candidates, as countless candidates are to be screened for multiple roles, adversely impacting the quality of recruitment. Manual screening of resumes is the most onerous part of recruiting, especially because 75 to 88 percent of the total resumes that are received for a role are of unqualified candidates. It is estimated that screening and shortlisting candidates for interviews take about 23 h or more of a recruiter's time just for a single hire [5].

Interviewing: An interview is an exchange of ideas, involving communication between the interviewer and the interviewee for finding information about the attitude, qualities, skills, experience, and prospects of a candidate accepting an offer in case of selection. Interviews can be either formal or informal and can be conducted face to face or over a telecon or through video conferencing [6]. Interviewing requires scheduling, rescheduling, cancellation of appointments, sending and sharing notes, sending reminders, and recommending resources for evaluation. The constant tracing, tracking, follow-up scheduling, rescheduling involving multiple candidates and multiple hiring managers is a very difficult and exhausting task for the recruiter.

Moreover, as jobs are becoming extremely technical and domain-specific, traditional forms of interviewing are no longer considered good enough to gauge a candidate's fitment. Multiple rounds of interviews, various psychological and psychometric tests have become a part of the recruitment process. Nonetheless, with the inclusion of these multiple steps, recruitment only becomes slow and more challenging. While the Applicant Tracking Software (ATS) and various other software have been in place for assisting the hiring teams, managing and coordinating with multiple stakeholders remains to be a prime challenge.

Selection and Offer: Selection is the process of picking the most suitable candidate for the job, out of all the qualified candidates that have cleared the multiple stages of the recruitment and selection process [7]. Once the candidates clear the multiple levels and reach the final stage of selection, the hiring manager is on the hook for zeroing down on the most suitable candidate from the qualified ones. The hiring decision is extremely important as any mistake at this point can ruin all the efforts thus far. Several aspects need to be taken into consideration apart from just the knowledge, expertise, and experience of the candidate. The candidates, cultural fit with the organization, and his expected stability at the job matter equally as much but are aspects that are difficult to predict and often escape the purview of even the most experienced recruiters, interviewers, and functional managers.

The final stage where the offer of appointment is laid out to the candidate holds as much importance or rather more as the acceptance of the offer and acknowledgment to join. Many companies experience a no-show on the date of joining and hence only when a candidate reports to work on the day of joining can the efforts of the hiring team be considered successful. However as there is no dearth of offers for high potential candidates, they are mostly contemplating multiple proposals at any given time. Gone are the days when a one size fits all approach could be applied to rolling out the employment terms. Candidates today demand personalized offers based on their aspirations and unique requirements. An organization's failure at providing an appealing compensation package can lead to the rejection of the employment proposal, pushing all the efforts back to zero. Organizations today should be prepared to roll out offers that are tweaked and personalized to the candidate's demands and expectations. This requires a thorough understanding of the international job market, salaries, and perks offered by the competition, being aware of the key motivators that candidates find appealing, and benchmarking remuneration packages against the best in the industry. The final terms of appointment should be alluring, fulfilling, and motivating enough to ensure a long-term engagement with the organization. Recruitment demands commitment in terms of time and resources, and a failed recruiting attempt is a huge loss to the organization. Yet, there are instances where, after chasing candidates through multiple stages of the hiring process, they drop out at the end due to an unattractive and non-compelling offer, leaving all efforts of the hiring team undone.

Onboarding: The process of introducing the new hire to the organization's culture and environment is referred to as Onboarding. With the acceptance of the offer by the candidate and formalization of the joining dates, the process of onboarding begins. Onboarding is a critical aspect of recruitment and retention of talent and requires proper planning coordination and implementation. Different organizations have differently designed onboarding processes, in some organizations, it is a one-day event while in others the time taken to complete onboarding could even extend up to 18 months. Undermining the importance of the Onboarding process can be one of the gravest mistakes that any organization commits. Research by the Work Institute based on 34,000 exit interviews, reveals that more than 40% of new hire's quit in the very first year of employment [8]. If the first impression is bad, it can damage the reputation and perception of the employer beyond repair. An ineffective onboarding process can lead to many issues including low employee morale, engagement, and confidence leading to poor performance, missed targets, and employee turnover [9]. With the employee turnover, recruitment requires to begin again from scratch. Employee onboarding is exacting as, in the initial phase of employment, employees require constant handholding and guidance to understand everything from the way of working, policies, and culture and hence it demands 24/7 assistance from the HR team. Comprehensive onboarding systems allow employees to succeed and flourish, while poorly designed ones become a disadvantage. For small hiring teams, dealing with the massive task of recruitment, in parallel with ensuring a smooth and seamless onboarding experience that demands round-the-clock support is almost unachievable.

Hiring undoubtedly is an effortful job and needs the support of technology to make it more manageable and concise. This is where innovations in technology and advancements in AI, targeting the automation and up-gradation of recruitment are a source of great relief. AI and machine learning are making their way into every aspect of recruitment, taking away the burden of repetitive tasks, restructuring processes, and providing employers with the capability to manage to hire more effectively and efficiently without having to involve a higher number of people. Organizations all across the globe have witnessed and acknowledged the power of AI to transform and revolutionize the entire hiring and recruiting space. As a result, businesses worldwide have expedited their plans of incorporating AI solutions to reform the process of recruitment.

Making Recruitment Smarter with AI

AI is ubiquitous, touching our lives at multiple points throughout the day. From accessing smartphones through face detection, sending autocorrected emails, conversing with Alexa, and Siri to navigating via google maps, AI touches our lives in ways beyond our cognition. Such is the power of AI that every business and function is welcoming the inclusion of AI into their systems and processes to infuse efficiency and effectiveness while eliminating mundane tasks.

Experts realize that AI can speed up the expensive, time-consuming, subjective, and reactive process of talent acquisition, and therefore HR managers and recruiters have taken the leap and embraced AI for ameliorating the entire hiring landscape. AI is transforming how businesses recruit, re-recruit, support, develop, retrain, train, and retain new and existing staff. AI has made its way into every stage, every step of the process of recruitment for all the right reasons (Fig. 14.1).

By screening the initial pool of applicants based on performance potential, to automating manual processes leading to reduction of the possibility of human error and prejudice, AI can significantly accelerate the recruitment processes. Companies are increasingly adopting AI to source qualified candidates and augment their ability to discover the right candidate at the right time.

AI can jump into action even before an open job position is advertised. With its ability to think and reason, AI can notify the right people with the precise skill sets about vacant positions to both active and passive candidates that fit the job requirements. Also, with the ability to understand synonymous words that applicants often use in resumes, in addition to simple key terms used for search, AI can identify

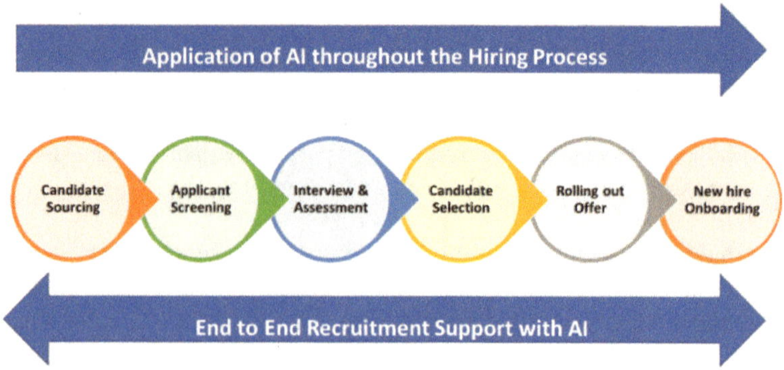

Fig. 14.1 AI application throughout the Hiring process [10]

the best fit of candidates for the occupation based on their skills and experience. AI can leverage data to predict and determine a candidate's possibility of accepting an offer, project expected performance results, and forecast expected tenure. AI software can sort more than 3 billion pages of data per day, leading to a significant reduction of the recruiter's workload. Also, the prospects sourced by AI algorithms, create a ready pool of candidates that have a high probability of clearing the recruitment process and accepting the offer [11].

The automation of the high-volume task of screening resumes through the application of AI frees up the recruiter's time and considerably reduces workload. In addition to matching basic job requirements with the information already present on resumes, AI screeners can pull up public data about the candidate from various social media platforms to derive a complete and more conclusive picture of the candidate. Besides AI can substantially reduce or almost eliminate human bias while assessing job applicants, making the process of screening more objective and data-driven. As a result, candidate screening solutions powered by AI are emerging as an important segment in the space of AI-powered recruiting, improving the overall quality of the screening process and hiring as such.

The inclusion of AI in candidate assessment can considerably augment the process. Selection can be made based on data instead of guesses and the interviewer's judgment. Utilizing AI for personality testing of candidates can help measure their cognitive ability and emotional intelligence. Traits such as agreeableness, consciousness, extroversion, neuroticism, and openness to experience that are otherwise difficult to quantify can also be measured with the help of AI assessment tools [12]. These traits can help predict how an individual would perform at work, collaborate, organize, be assertive, and be innovative in addition to being open to new ideas and learning. Gaining an insight into a candidate's emotional intelligence is important to predict their cultural fit within an organization.

The use of AI-powered applications for interviewing can accelerate the rate at which organizations can evaluate potential candidates while creating a highly engaging applicant experience at the same time. Chatbot software can support continued engagement with candidates guiding them throughout the application and interview process, providing feedback on their application acceptance and probable hiring status, in cases of both selection and rejection [12]. Chatbots are increasingly being used for scheduling interviews with viable applicants, offering continuous support, providing immediate replies to queries and inquiries, and reflecting the brand and voice of the organization.

AI makes it possible to remove social, performance, or personal bias from the process of interviewing, making it fair and robust. With AI, data from prior employees performing similar tasks can be collated and used to prepare tailored questions that the hiring manager can utilize during interviews to avoid subjectivity. The potential elimination of a good candidate can be evaded by using a pre-screening process that can remove interviewer biases. The recruiting industry today is progressively adopting automated video interviews that evaluate a candidate's communications skills and also provide a behavioral analysis to predict job performance [10].

Adoption of game mechanics such as achievement and competition for assessing personality traits and reactions to different situations provides a better estimate of a candidate's fitment for a role [13]. The application of AI through the Interview and assessment process makes the hiring decision more informed, easy, and faster for the candidates, recruiters, and hiring managers alike.

Post selection, AI tools with predictive intelligence offer insights on a candidate's past employment, salary expectations, and offer acceptance behavior. This information is vital as it can help organizations improve the offer-to-join ratio while lowering hiring costs by almost up to 50% [14]. AI and Catboats have made it possible to automate the entire process of rolling out offer letters, receiving acknowledgment, and providing instant replies to candidate queries.

Once an offer gets accepted, onboarding kicks off from the first day of reporting. Onboarding is vital, for making a lasting impression that would decide a new hire's willingness to have a long and fulfilling career with the organization or otherwise. Taking the help of AI at this stage can turn around things in the organization's favor. The inefficiencies in the process of onboarding can be overcome with the implementation of AI Chatbots. Onboarding bots or personal AI assistants integrate with HR management systems to act as a new hire's guide to the new workplace, facilitating a smooth and enriching onboarding experience [10]. AI can automate arduous account setups, track the progress of tasks, prompt responses, and answer questions instantly that most new hires are bound to have. Basic questions with regard to setting up an email account connecting to the office Wi-Fi, setting up data security protocols, policies, and more can be managed seamlessly by AI chatbots. Besides creating an engaging experience for new employees by addressing FAQs and with the ability to learn, AI software can be programmed and upgraded simultaneously to address new queries. Furthermore, AI with Neuro-Linguistic Programming can analyze and extract quality insights from documented feedback about the onboarding, usually running into thousands of pages, to design and implement initiatives to improve the current process.

The HR fraternity is realizing the power of AI and its ability to renovate and revolutionize the whole function of HRM, resulting in an ever-increasing demand for AI technology for automation of the end-to-end recruitment process. The market today is flooded with AI-Powered enterprise solutions that can provide thrust and momentum to businesses. McKinsey Gold survey (2019) suggested a 25% year-on-year increase in the adoption of AI in business operations, and the IDC forecast predicts the worldwide revenue of AI market's crossing 300 billion USD by 2024, the future is certainly going to be dominated by AI [15]. As a result, innovators in the field of technology are vigorously working on creating AI solutions for businesses of all kinds. AI packages are offered with different functionalities at different costs. Any business irrespective of its size, sector, or industry today has access to AI solutions that can fit in their budgets and help them achieve their business aspirations.

Key Benefits of Adopting AI in Recruiting

AI supports and strengthens every aspect of Recruitment and the overall hiring process in numerous ways. AI-Powered recruitment solutions can benefit businesses on a strategic level. The key benefits of AI inclusion can be sorted under the following categories[16] (Fig. 14.2).

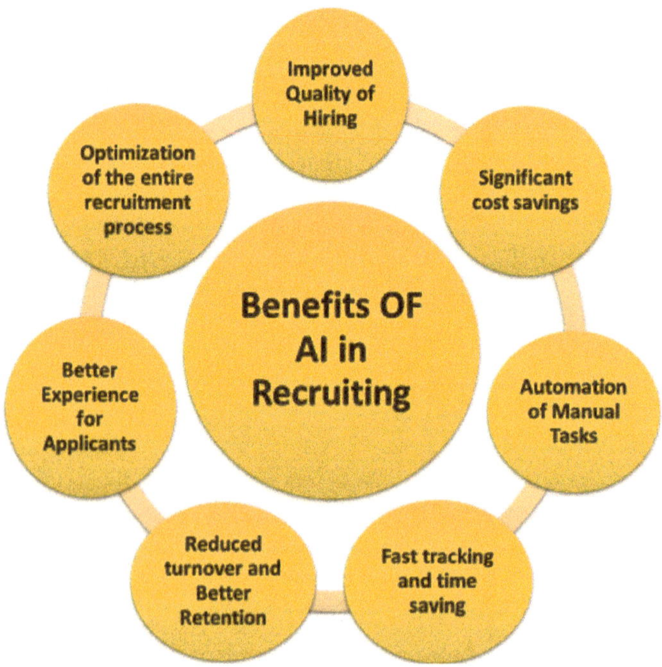
Improved Quality of Hiring
Significant cost savings
Automation of Manual Tasks
Fast tracking and time saving
Reduced turnover and Better Retention
Better Experience for Applicants
Optimization of the entire recruitment process
Benefits OF AI in Recruiting

Fig. 14.2 Key benefits of AI in recruitment [17]

Better hiring quality: AI's capability of finding a more precise match between applicants and vacant positions significantly improves the accuracy of the hiring process leading to a mutually fulfilling engagement for both applicants and the employer. Also, better matching lowers the risk of candidate turnover, preventing candidate exit midway through the hiring process.

Cost-effective hiring: Perhaps one of the most important benefits of incorporating AI power into recruitment is the significant reduction in cost per hire. As "time is money" AI shortens the time taken from filling in a few open positions to accomplishing volume hiring. AI substantially reduces valuable operational time and resource costs. Leading global corporations have been able to achieve a reduction in cost per hire by almost up to 30% with AI [19].

Automation of the hiring Process: AI solutions enable the end-to-end automation of the hiring process. With AI candidates can be pre-screened by administering pre-recorded video interviews. Scheduling software allows candidates the flexibility to schedule and reschedules themselves based on availability requiring minimal intervention from the hiring team. With mobile recruiting apps recruitment can be done on the go, without location and time constraints. AI can create and maintain talent communities, enlisting millions of applicants that form a database and a pipeline of instantly accessible qualified candidates. Implementation of Candidate relationship management system (CRM), and its integration with other tools such as scheduling software, campus recruiting tools can allow recruitment to run on autopilot [18].

AI Saves Time: Automation of repetitive mundane tasks with AI results in significant time saving, allowing recruiters to focus on other important responsibilities. Workflow automation streamlines processes and makes them efficient. Tasks such as screening resumes and providing round-the-clock support to candidates can be put on autopilot saving substantial effort and time.

Better Retention and Reduced Turnover: The analytics to retention and attrition data using AI tools can provide meaningful insights into the reasons behind turnover. This information can be used to design interventions for improving the overall employee experience. Fraud detection, absence, and accident prediction with AI can prove highly beneficial in proactively driving initiatives to evade any mishaps.

Improved candidate satisfaction: An organization's reputation as an employer is a key aspect for attracting and retaining high-quality talent. Often, non-responsiveness and a sluggish recruitment process end up damaging an employer's name and image. Faster processing of resumes and timely updates on application status leads to improved candidate satisfaction and a better outlook toward the organization.

Optimization of the Hiring Process: AI can help organizations put their hiring act together. AI software can be used to optimize parts or the entire process of recruitment. Businesses can pick and choose AI software depending on the aspects of their current process they wish to address and enhance. Automation and optimization through AI allow hiring teams the bandwidth to focus their efforts on critical issues, enabling effective use of their time and resources.

Top AI Software for Recruitment

AI offers multiple benefits, and every organization today wants to take advantage of its power. However, the adoption of AI is a means to an end and not the end in itself. Organizations should acquire a profound understanding of the results they wish to achieve by the adoption of this technology. The current market is swamped with software solution providers, offering various AI tools for recruitment that offer different features and functionalities. Some AI solutions upgrade the entire recruitment process, while others focus on a single or specific aspect of recruitment. AI solutions are investment-heavy and therefore should be initiated only post an appropriate cost–benefit analysis. Listed below are the top 10 AI-powered recruiting software, their key features, and renowned global organizations that have benefitted from their implementation [20] (Table 14.1).

1. **AI for business continuity, crisis management, and as a source of competitive advantage.**

   Besides the numerous advantages that AI offers, in terms of cost and time saving, organizations have lately realized its power to ensure business continuity and manage the crisis. With AI companies were able to function seamlessly through the pandemic, proving its legitimacy as a source of competitive advantage. The coronavirus outbreak in the year 2020 was without a doubt the most difficult crisis the world witnessed in recent times. It drastically hit business operations globally, leading to a freeze on hiring in many cases and extreme reductions in recruitment budgets. Being cost-effective and efficient with recruitment initiatives became all the more critical for the hiring teams during this period. However, as mobility became a major challenge, for both employers and candidates, recruiters were left with no option but to move to Google meet or Zoom interviews for assessing candidates. This move did not really help, as for recruiters to sit through one Zoom call after another, throughout the day was not a productive utilization of time, and it led to the realization that Artificial Intelligence and machine learning could be a game-changer in this scenario. With hiring teams specifically strapped for time and resources, leaning on to automation and smart AI technology became the need of the hour. The pandemic accelerated the adoption of AI recruitment solutions globally, as it became a matter of survival.

   While AI has proven its supremacy as a technology that has the potential to completely change the way businesses function for good, its true power was realized during the pandemic. With lockdowns and restrictions in place for both employers and candidates, recruiters had to look toward AI to source smartly, recruit effectively, and make quality hires while being cost-effective. The ability of AI-powered software to source, pre-screen, screen, schedule, assess, interview, select, and onboard even remote candidates effectively, helped businesses recruit quality candidates, faster and efficiently within restricted budgets. A study by The Sage Group suggests that 24% of businesses have already begun

Table 14.1 List of top 10 AI recruiting software

Top AI recruiting software			
Software	Suitable for	Key Features	Clients
XOR	Large organizations	• AI chatbot by XOR can handle internal and External Candidates • Customizable questions and scoring and sorting applicants on autopilot	Delta Dallas, Targul de Cariere, 4 M Logistics
Hiretual	All types and sizes of companies,	• Focuses mainly on sourcing • Enables exploring beyond main platforms and internal databases	Tangocard, APPTIO, CORNERSTONE
Eightfold	Large organizations Enterprise clients with 2,000 + employees	• AI Powered talent intelligence platform • Reviewing millions of candidate profiles within seconds	TATA Communications, Air Asia, Netapp, BAYER
Paradox	High-volume hiring	• Olivia, a conversational artificial intelligence agent, puts candidates in control of the conversation	Wendy's, Visiting Angles, Koch Trucking
AmazingHiring	High volume tech hiring	• Can aggregate professional backgrounds of technical candidates from over 70 different sources	Intellectsoft, Deutsche Bank, Hays, ABBYY

(continued)

Table 14.1 (continued)

Top AI recruiting software

Software	Suitable for	Key Features	Clients
SeekOut	Large to small recruiting teams & Agencies	• Many variants of artificial intelligence within a search engine • Database of 500 million talent profiles	Rover, Twitter, VMware, Wellpath
Humanly	Medium-sized companies	• Integrates with the main ATS • Focuses on diversity hiring • Integrates sourcing sites with ATS	ARMOIRE, BPM, Swiss Monkey, and Dasro
HireVue	Large Enterprises	• Can source, screen, and schedule candidates, saving time and cost	Unilever, Cathay Pacific, Randstad, G4S, Foxtel Group
Pymetrics	Companies with 5,000 + candidate pool	• Leverages gamification, behavioral science, and AI technology • Assessment of personality fit, characteristics, and behavioral traits using Video Games	PWC, BCG, Accenture, McDonald's, ANZ, Colgate-Palmolive
LOXO	All sizes, all industries Individual consultants & Small recruitment teams	• Full-fledged recruitment CRM • Maintain an updated database of more than 530 million professionals	BVOH Ngrowth Amazon

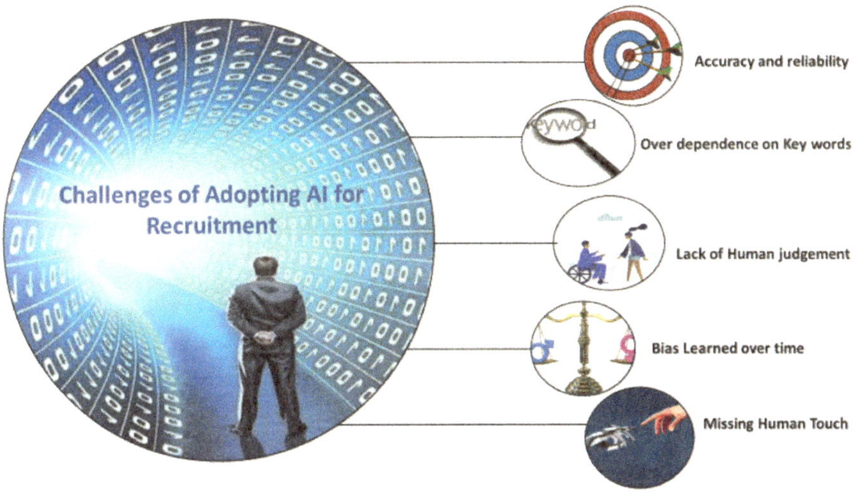

Fig. 14.3 Challenges of adopting AI for recruitment

using AI for talent acquisition, with 56% of executives planning to adopt AI technology in the coming year [21].

The right AI solution without a doubt is an important source of competitive advantage and that explains the rush for its adoption by companies worldwide. However, for organizations climbing on the bandwagon without truly understanding what AI can deliver and matching its capabilities with their business needs would only lead to complicating things as against the expectation of simplification and optimization (Fig. 14.3).

2. **The flip side of adopting AI for Recruitment**

   There is enough evidence to support the role of AI in transforming and enhancing the function of recruitment and the overall hiring process. However, in this haste to include and implement AI in recruitment, it is very likely to overlook some of the shortcomings that this technology suffers from. AI is not foolproof, and it does come with its fair share of challenges [22].

Reliability and Accuracy issues: Though AI has become the Holy Grail, the truth is that it is not perfect. It suffers from issues related to accuracy and reliability. Different formatting or resume styles can confuse AI systems. There is a high possibility that a well-qualified applicant might not make it through the AI screening system due to the use of a different format or a minor issue such as an unconventional style of bullet points used in the resume.

Over dependence on Key Words: AI uses keywords to scan through various job portals and databases. Someone with an understanding of how AI systems are programmed has a clear advantage over others. With their understanding of the system, they acquire the ability to trick the system and camouflage their candidature as a good fit using the keywords that the AI programs have been fed. While in reality there may be far better candidates that may not make it through the pre-programmed AI search.

Lack of Human judgement: Organizations looking to diversify their workforce may not benefit from AI. Experiences in a certain field are not always the most important criteria for candidates' expected performance in another. Candidates with atypical work experience may make a good fit for a job role based on their personality, character, personal interests, ethnicity, and work ethics. Using AI in such hiring scenarios can prove to be of no use, as these decisions mandate real human judgment and not intelligence that is artificial.

Bias learned over time: While the popular perception is that AI promotes unbiased hiring, in reality AI systems learn through past trends and patterns and can therefore pick up and include partial past decisions made based on age, gender, ethnicity, or alma mater of the candidates. This problem though fixable should be kept in consideration by the organizations looking to automate hiring using AI. Amazon.com had to scrap a secret recruiting tool that was observed to show bias against women [23]. Developers of AI systems must take necessary steps to eliminate such forms of human error and ensure these biases do not creep into the AI algorithms.

The missing Human touch: AI after all is human-like, but not human and cannot, therefore, connect with people as well as a real person can. Though AI can make hiring more effective and simpler, it may not be able to communicate as effectively. AI-powered chatbots can make communication feel impersonal to both the candidates and hiring managers. The hiring managers may feel detached from the process, and candidates may not be satisfied and convinced with the generic messages received from catboats. This limitation, however, can be overcome if hiring managers utilize their time saved as a result of process automation, on getting to know the candidates better. AI should be applied to automate tasks and not jobs, leaving important aspects like interviewing and final selection to experienced Managers. AI adoption should be a well-thought strategic decision, with a strong understanding of desired outcomes.

In the end, given the enormous task of recruitment and volume hiring, the pros of using AI in recruitment clearly outweigh the cons and hence many high-performing recruitment teams are already leveraging the power of artificial intelligence while many others are in the process of adopting AI. The popular belief surely seems to be that the drawbacks of AI are trivial and the positives are definitely worth the risk.

Conclusion

AI is the future, and its dominance in every field including Recruitment is only bound to increase. Automation of the recruitment process saves time and cost allowing recruiters to focus on other more critical tasks. In a matter of time, we would witness AI take over the entire recruitment landscape, just like every other aspect of our lives. The traditional hiring practices will soon be replaced with AI-powered hiring.

However, while adopting AI, organizations should be mindful of addressing candidate concerns around bias and discrimination and that of its employees harboring the fear of Job cuts. AI and machine learning should be brought in to eliminate the burden of boring and repetitive tasks and not for shredding jobs. The success of AI implementation would largely depend on the way employees receive it and therefore addressing their insecurities and taking them into confidence would be extremely vital. Besides, acknowledging and accepting that AI does suffer from a few challenges and working around these concerns would be important to mitigate risks while making the most out of its implementation. Eventually though, with continuous efforts from technology experts, solutions would be found to address the minor inadequacies of AI and Machine learning. The principal challenge for AI experts in the future would be designing machines that can learn to emote like humans or rather we could say the Humanization of AI is the need of the hour. The Amalgamation of Artificial Intelligence and Emotional Intelligence is what the future demands and would be interesting to witness. The world of recruiting is moving beyond AI, demanding EI enabled AI solutions.

References

1. A Look at the Most Used Terminology Around Artificial Intelligence. https://interestingengineering.com/a-look-at-the-most-used-terminology-around-artificial-intelligence. Accessed 19 July 2021
2. Artificial Intelligence—Google Books. https://www.google.co.in/books/edition/ARTIFICIAL_INTELLIGENCE/v_jhDAAAQBAJ?hl=en&gbpv=1&dq=artificial+intelligence+meaning&printsec=frontcover. Accessed 19 July 2021
3. Recruitment Process—Tutorialspoint. https://www.tutorialspoint.com/recruitment_and_selection/recruitment_process.htm. Accessed 19 July 2021
4. Recruiting: What is sourcing? https://www.shrm.org/resourcesandtools/tools-and-samples/hr-qa/pages/whatissourcing.aspx. Accessed 19 July 2021
5. AI For Recruiting: A Definitive Guide For HR Professionals | Ideal. https://ideal.com/ai-recruiting/. Accessed 22 July 2021
6. Recruitment Interviews—Tutorialspoint. https://www.tutorialspoint.com/recruitment_and_selection/recruitment_interviews.htm. Accessed 19 July 2021
7. What is Selection?—Tutorialspoint. https://www.tutorialspoint.com/recruitment_and_selection/what_is_selection.htm. Accessed 22 July 2021
8. AI in HR. https://www.adaface.com/blog/ai-in-hr/. Accessed 22 July 2021
9. The drastic drawbacks of an ineffective onboarding process—DronaHQ. https://www.dronahq.com/the-drastic-drawbacks-of-an-ineffective-onboarding-process/. Accessed 22 July 2021
10. How to Succeed with AI in Recruiting | HR Technologist. https://www.hrtechnologist.com/articles/digital-transformation/how-to-succeed-with-ai-in-recruiting/. Accessed 22 July 2021
11. AI Passive Candidate Sourcing: A Powerful Approach to Hiring | CEIPAL. https://www.ceipal.com/ai-passive-candidate-sourcing-a-powerful-approach-to-hiring/. Accessed 22 July 2021
12. How Is Artificial Intelligence Changing the Recruiting Process? https://www.mbassett.com/blog/how-is-artificial-intelligence-changing-the-recruiting-process. Accessed 22 July 2021
13. How to Use AI and Gamification in Hiring for Effective Recruitment. https://blogs.fireflies.ai/ai-and-gamification-in-hiring/. Accessed 22 July 2021
14. HRtech startup HireSure.ai is using AI and blockchain to address hiring inefficiencies. https://yourstory.com/2020/09/hrtech-startup-hiresureai-ai-blockchain-hiring/amp. Accessed 22 July 2021

15. How Emerging Demands Of AI-Powered Solutions Help Gain Momentum of Businesses. https://www.entrepreneur.com/article/359159. Accessed 23 July 2021
16. AI for Recruiting: Everything you Need to Know—Dashbouquet. https://dashbouquet.com/blog/artificial-intelligence/ai-for-recruiting-everything-you-need-to-know. Accessed 24 July 2021
17. How to Succeed with AI in Recruiting | HR Technologist. https://www.hrtechnologist.com/articles/digital-transformation/how-to-succeed-with-ai-in-recruiting/. Accessed 25 July 2021
18. 6 Ways to Automate Recruiting Processes. https://yello.co/blog/6-ways-automate-recruiting-processes/. Accessed 24 July 2021.
19. How AI recruitment software can reduce the cost of hiring. https://otomeyt.ai/blog/can-ai-recruitment-software-reduce-the-cost-of-hiring/. Accessed 24 July 2021
20. The Top 12 Best AI Recruiting Tools - March 2021 | SelectSoftware Reviews. https://www.selectsoftwarereviews.com/buyer-guide/ai-recruiting. Accessed 23 July 2021
21. How artificial intelligence is being used to recruit and onboard talent. https://digiday.com/marketing/ai-is-being-used-to-recruit-and-onboard-talent/. Accessed 24 July 2021
22. Weighing in on the pros and cons of AI in HR recruitment. https://www.jobstreet.com.sg/en/cms/employer/weighing-pros-cons-ai-hr-recruitment/. Accessed 25 July 2021
23. To recruit top talent, we need emotionally intelligent AI | Cybersecurity & Technology News | Secure Futures | Kaspersky. https://www.kaspersky.com/blog/secure-futures-magazine/ai-emotionally-intelligent-recruitment/37863/. Accessed 27 July 2021

Chapter 15
Technology Versus Tradition: Game Theoretic Model for Human-Animal Conflict in the Evolution of Digital Society

Saurabh Shanu

Introduction

Many complicated jobs have become relatively easy to grasp and work on because of advancements in many disciplines of science and related technology. Wildlife conservation is one such field [30]. Many technological activities have been introduced, particularly in and near Protected Areas (PAs), with the goal of preserving natural species [4]. Placement of camera traps, line transects utilizing mobile and digital compass, drone photography, bird trackers on electric wires and so on are only a few examples [31]. All of them are designed to estimate animal density and abundance or to protect wild animals from manmade or natural threats [16].

Conservation efforts are currently concentrated mostly in and around the PAs. Human settlements, including villages and agricultural fields, are found on the outskirts of these PAs [11]. As a result, these places become hotspots of human-animal conflict. These regions are not only becoming a hotspot, but they are also underdeveloped and have a conventional approach to wild animals [8]. Following these methods, the people frequently support as well as criticize the technical procedures used in the forest for conservation. For wildlife stakeholders, moving in line with people's traditional and daily behaviours is a major concern [7].

Scholarships conducted one such study, which demonstrates both support for and devaluation of technology techniques in PAs. To begin, while discussing downgrading activities, the greatest example that can be given is video traps for wildlife monitoring in peripheral zones [15]. Villager's customary traditions led to the removal and destruction of cameras in the area, according to studies. Open deification, cow grazing, mythical rites of being seen and so on are examples of these

S. Shanu (✉)
Department of Virtualization, School of Computer Science and Engineering, University of Petroleum and Energy Studies, Dehradun, Uttarakhand 248007, India
e-mail: sshanu@ddn.upes.ac.in

A. Choudhury et al. (eds.), *Evolution of Digitized Societies Through Advanced Technologies*, Advanced Technologies and Societal Change,
https://doi.org/10.1007/978-981-19-2984-7_15

traditional activities [14]. Second, when it comes to how people have reacted to the employment of technology for wildlife conservation, the greatest example to provide is the use of electrocution around agricultural fields to prevent animals from entering the fields and thereby preserving crops and animal lives [13].

The above explanation demonstrates how traditional behaviours and technological deployments must be actively understood in tandem. The chapter aims to create a model over a hypothetical landscape in order to simulate the conditions surrounding a protected area, which might be utilized to deploy technology solutions in harmony with local activities. Locals pose a significant danger to the protection of wild species, thus maintaining this equilibrium is critical [19]. The model developed because of this research is an applied mathematical model that considers the many levels of interaction between traditional practices and technological deployment in order to produce an interaction graph [10]. These interaction graphs would be used to create a network of activities and then identify the clusters within the network in order to identify essential and crucial activities as well as the places where they should be carried out.

The conflict between technological deployment and traditional behaviours is viewed as a core issue with the network's underlying clusters. Detecting the aforementioned would be extremely beneficial in understanding why disputes arise and how to resolve those [23]. In this chapter, the method to finding a solution to the given problem is entirely based on applied mathematics and computation theories.

The preceding discussion aids in the identification of two distinct sets of points or clusters. The first cluster has been dubbed the cooperative cluster, in which all local solutions are categorized, and the second cluster has been dubbed the defecting cluster, in which all local practices that have been downgraded are retained. This information, as well as how to strike a balance between the two, would be extremely useful in identifying the best strategies and planning for the deployment of technology solutions for animal conservation.

The following parts go through the hypothetical landscape, the materials and techniques utilized, the methodology suggested in the work, the findings produced using the created model, the discussion of the results, and the work's conclusion and limits.

Hypothetical Landscape

A hypothetical landscape is examined for the sake of the suggested model in the work, as illustrated in Fig. 15.1. The scene depicts a forest area, hamlet areas, agricultural fields, forest perimeter regions, and a villagers' pilgrimage place located within the forest. The bulk of contradictory arguments arises in these regions, which is why these components have been considered. There might be a variety of additional elements that influence conflict sites, but in order to keep the model simple and provide a basic computational template, it was believed that just these areas are essential.

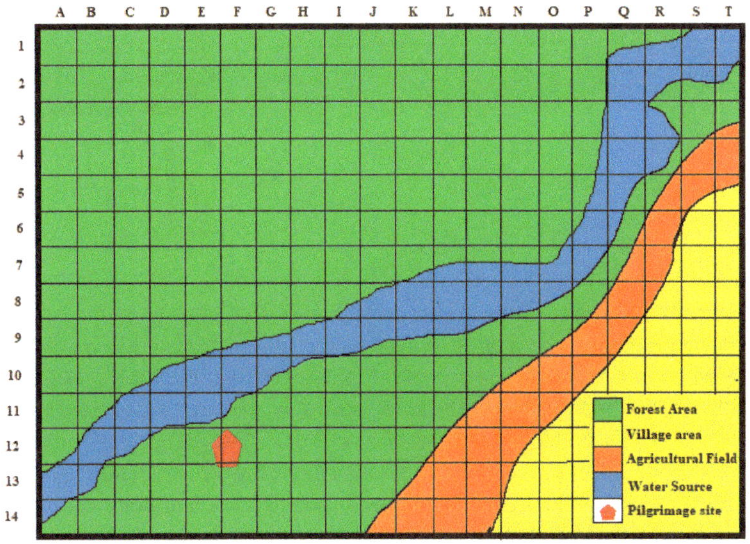

Fig. 15.1 Hypothetical landscape

The entire terrain is split into comparable geographical grids, each with an area of n hectares, for comprehending the landscape characteristics. Each grid's nomenclature is provided in the style of a chess system. In the imagined landscape, the pilgrimage site, for example, is divided into four grids: $E12$, $E13$, $F12\&F14$. A collection of crucial grids is extracted as set Z using the proposed terminology, as follows:

$$Z = \left\{\left\{a_{ij}\right\}\right\} \cup \left\{b_{pk}\right\} | i \in \{D, E, F, G, H, I, J, K, L, M\}, j \in \{9, 10, 11, 12, 13, 14, 15\}, \\ p \in \{N, P, Q, R, S, T\} \& k \in \{2, 3, 4, 5, 6, 7, 8, 9\}|$$

where, a_{ij} and b_{pk} represent the grids with the nomenclature ij and pk, respectively.

Materials and Concepts

Modelling the competing and enhancing interactions of traditional practices with technology advancements for animal conservation is a significant issue in this work. Initially, game theory is employed in order to comprehend this. A game G may be described as a three-tuple consisting of a set of players, a set of strategies, and a set of related payoffs [9]. As a result, a game G is

$$G = (P, S, \zeta)$$

		P1	
		C	D
P2	C	(3, 3)	(0, 5)
	D	(5, 0)	(1, 1)

Fig. 15.2 Payoff matrix of 2-persons prisoner's dilemma game

where P represents the set of players, S represents the set of strategies and ζ represents the associated payoffs. The payoff represents the scores achieved by each player in the set P while using any of the strategies in the set S. Because the goal of this work is to better understand cooperation and defection, a two-person prisoner's dilemma game was chosen to simulate the interactions [28].

The prisoner's dilemma is a non-cooperative game theory case that shows why two reasonable persons would refuse to cooperate even if it was in their best interests to do so. A two-person prisoner's dilemma game features two participants, as the name implies. At the same time, the game's strategy set is limited to only two options: cooperation *(C)* and defection *(D)*. As a result, each participant in the prisoner's dilemma game can either collaborate or defect, earning a score depending on his own and the opponent's choices [12]. As a result, Fig. 15.2 depicts the payoff matrix that may be used to award a score to players based on the sort of strategy they apply.

The next computational ideas are developed from graph theory after deciding on the scores over interactions acquired by game theory. A graph may be described as a two-tuple consisting of a set of vertices and a set of edges [3] with the following properties:

$$G'' = (V, E)$$

where V denotes the set of vertices and E denotes the set of edges obtained by adjacency of vertices in the set V. The presence of an edge between any two vertices of the vertex set indicates that those two vertices interact [6]. These interactions are used in this chapter to better understand how vertices and their underlying edges are represented.

Cliques are one of the most important ideas developed from graph theory. Every vertex in a clique is linked to every other vertex. An *n*-clique is a clique with n vertices in which each vertex has no more than *(n-1)* edges [25]. Figure 15.3 depicts a graph as well as the clique that exists inside it.

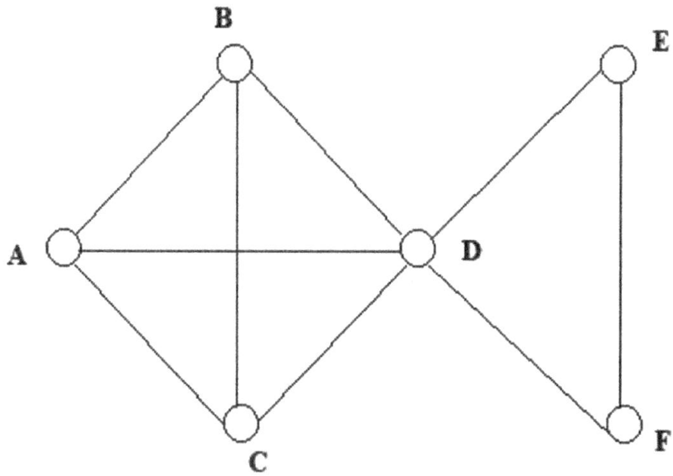

Fig. 15.3 A graph with cliques

Table 15.1 Cliques obtained from graph G" of Fig. 15.3

k-clique	Vertices forming k-clique
4-clique	{A, B, C, D}
3-clique	{A, B, C}, {B, C, D}, {A, C, D}, {D, E, F}
2-clique	{A, B}, {A, C}, {A, D}, {B, C}, {B, D}, {C, D}, {D, E}, {D, F}, {E, F}
1-clique	{A, B, C, D, E, F}

In Fig. 15.3, a graph G'' with 6 vertices and 9 vertices which can be written as $G'' = \{\{A, B, C, D, E, F\}, \{AB, AC, AD, BC, BD, CD, DE, DF, EF\}\}$ is represented. In the same graph, G", cliques can be identified which are shown in Table 15.1.

Clusters are discovered over the network generated by the resulting graphs after gaining knowledge of the cliques in the proposed complex system. These clusters are essentially a group of network vertices that have certain common characteristics and are more likely to be grouped together [5]. Weight centralities are utilized to identify the clusters. The structure of a network determines the centrality metrics [17]. The usage of weight centralities is discussed in the algorithm that follows.

```
Algorithm 1: Centrality_to_cluster
//Input: Network through the weighted graph G(V, E)
//Output: Clusters in the network
Declaration Section
        k, i as integer
        Record, V as set of vertices
Procedure Section
        For k = 0 to 5
            For i = 0 to |V|-1
                If w(Vi, Vi+1) = k
                    Record(k) = Record(k) U { Vi, Vi+1}
                End if
            End for
        End For

Result Section
        Set/Cluster of point showing clusters in the network based on weights.
```

Methodology

The goal of the research presented in this chapter is to develop a fundamental computational model that would maintain a balance between locals' traditional practices and modern deployments for animal protection. Initially, T is obtained as a set of conventional behaviours such that

$$T = \{T_1, T_2, T_3\}$$

where T_1 signifies open deification, T_2 signifies cattle grazing and T_3 signifies ceremonial activities. There might be many more components in the set T, but just three have been examined for the sake of presenting a model. According to the author of the chapter, increasing the number of items in T will simply increase the number of variables while having no effect on the suggested calculations. Similarly, T' is a set of technology deployments that includes

$$T' = \{A_1, A_2, A_3\}$$

where A_1 signifies camera trapping, A_2 signifies smart patrolling and A_3 signifies animal detection fences. As aforementioned, there may be more deployments; however, for the sake of modelling this would increase the number of variables while maintaining the calculations.

Following that a game between the components of T and the elements of T' is modelled in the work. The interaction of the elements of T between themselves is considered to be cooperative in character, and the same is assumed for the elements of T'. As a result, the three distinct interaction equations and their payoffs may be mapped as follows:

$$\zeta_{ij} = \zeta_{T_i(C,D),A_j(C,D)} \forall i \in \{1, 2, 3\} \text{ and } j \in \{1, 2, 3\}$$
$$\zeta_{ii} = \zeta_{T_i(C,D),T_i(C,D)} = (3, 3) \forall i \in \{1, 2, 3\}$$
$$\zeta_{jj} = \zeta_{A_j(C,D),A_j(C,D)} = (3, 3) \forall i \in \{1, 2, 3\}$$

The scores of each interaction are calculated by utilizing game theory to model the various sets of interactions. After getting these ratings, the weights of the edges in a weighted graph are calculated using the scores [22]. The weighted graph is created by combining traditional techniques with technological technologies to create a set of vertices. Thus for the interaction graph *G'*, the set of vertices is obtained as

$$V = T \cup T' = \{T_1, T_2, T_3, A_1, A_2, A_3\}$$

moreover, the set of edges is obtained as

$$\begin{aligned} E &= \{T \times T\} \cup \{T' \times T'\} \cup \{T \times T'\} \\ &= \{T_1T_2, T_1T_3, T_2T_3, A_1A_2, A_2A_3, A_1A_3, T_1A_1, T_1A_2, \\ &T_1A_3, T_2A_1, T_2A_2, T_2A_3, T_3A_1, T_3A_2, T_3A_3\} \end{aligned}$$

Each edge is given a weight depending on the payoffs achieved by the technical aspects through game theory interaction modelling. When there are intra-set interactions, the weights are freely modified with the payoffs on any element since it has no influence on the net weight because all outcomes are equal (3, 3).

After obtaining the graph, a network is created that represents the interaction of the proposed model's underlying parameters. Over the resulting network, the weight centrality is applied. The vertices are sorted by the weights they face in the analysis. The study shows a clustering of the vertices and therefore a method for cluster creation in a network utilizing Algorithm 1 stated previously. The clusters that develop have certain common vertices that are acquired and utilized for planning and strategizing purposes.

Results

Before moving on to the results, it's important to note that the remainder of the study focuses solely on the key grids indicated as *Z* in the suggested model. All interactions will take place only in those grids, and stringent forest regulations must be obeyed in the other grids. The interactions between the components of *T* and *T'* are discovered by treating each pair of *E* in the specified graph as the two players in the prisoner's dilemma game, as previously stated. The reward obtained by the technological components in each game is shown in Table 15.2.

Table 15.2 Payoff matrix for the interaction between elements of *T* and *T'*

Player 1	Player 2	Payoff
T_1 (D)	A_1 (C)	(5, 0)
T_1 (D)	A_2 (C)	(5, 0)
T_1 (C)	A_3 (C)	(3, 3)
T_2 (D)	A_1 (C)	(5, 0)
T_2 (C)	A_2 (D)	(0, 5)
T_2 (D)	A_3 (C)	(5, 0)
T_3 (C)	A_1 (C)	(3, 3)
T_3 (D)	A_2 (C)	(5, 0)
T_3 (C)	A_3 (D)	(0, 5)

Table 15.3 Cliques in the network obtained from the graph in Fig. 15.4

k-cliques	Vertices of the 6 clique
6-clique	$\{T_1, T_2, T_3, A_1, A_2, A_3\}$

It should be noticed that the reward for self-interaction between the members of the set *T* and *T'* is (3, 3).

After collecting the scores for each interaction, the weights of the weighted graph produced by considering all elements of *T* and *T'* as vertices are connected with the scores. Figure 15.4 depicts the resulting graph.

The cliques in the graph are found using the graph analysis [18] shown in Fig. 15.4. Getting the cliques is useful for figuring out how each element interacts with the others and what the greatest level of interaction is. Only the largest clique is retrieved as *n*-cliques from the proposed network for modelling purposes, where *n* is the highest potential degree of interaction that may occur in the network. Table 15.3 shows the cliques that develop in the network generated from Fig. 15.4's graph.

Following the discovery of the network's largest clique, method 1 is used to find the network's clusters based on the weights. Weights are used to split the clusters, and as seen in Fig. 15.4, there are three different weights, indicating that there are three separate clusters. Table 15.4 shows the many clusters that have developed, as well as the various interactions that belong to the clusters. Intra-set interactions are not investigated for cluster formation to maintain the model self-sustaining.

The knowledge acquired about clusters for the proposed model may be represented graphically as shown in Fig. 15.5.

Discussion

The findings of the model provided in this chapter show a very basic computational template for understanding the connections between various components of technology deployment and locals' traditional behaviours. Local opposition is

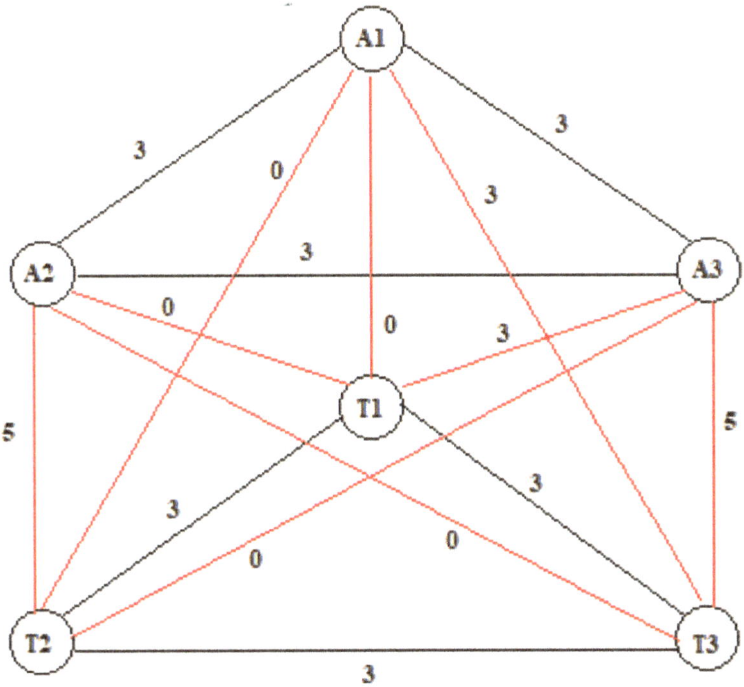

Fig. 15.4 Weighted graph obtained by modelling the interaction between the elements of *T* and *T'*

Table 15.4 Clusters formed in the network

Cluster name	Weight	Cluster interactions	Cluster vertices
C1	W = 0	$\{(T_2, A_1), (T_1, A_2), (T_2, A_3), (T_1, A_1)\}$	$\{T_1, T_2, A_1, A_2, A_3\}$
C2	W = 3	$\{(T_3, A_1), (T_1, A_3)\}$	$\{T_1, T_3, A_1, A_3\}$
C3	W = 5	$\{(T_2, A_2), (T_3, A_3)\}$	$\{T_2, T_3, A_2, A_3\}$

one of the problems that arises with the implementation of technology for animal protection [27]. The suggested model's application provides a deterministic method for computing a state of equilibrium for the successful deployment of technology components in wildlife conservation. As a result, the study focuses on how to organize technology deployment such that even locals are on board with its use and applications.

The suggested model is based on some of the most fundamental ideas in applied mathematics, such as game theory, graph theory, clusters and so on [22]. The challenge of comprehending the interplay between the parts of contradictions is initially accomplished using game theory [2]. The technical aspect is given a score for each pair of interactions, with 0 being the lowest and 5 being the highest. A score of 0 indicates that the technical element is subject to a high level of defection or relegation from the residents, whilst a score of 5 indicates that, while the element is

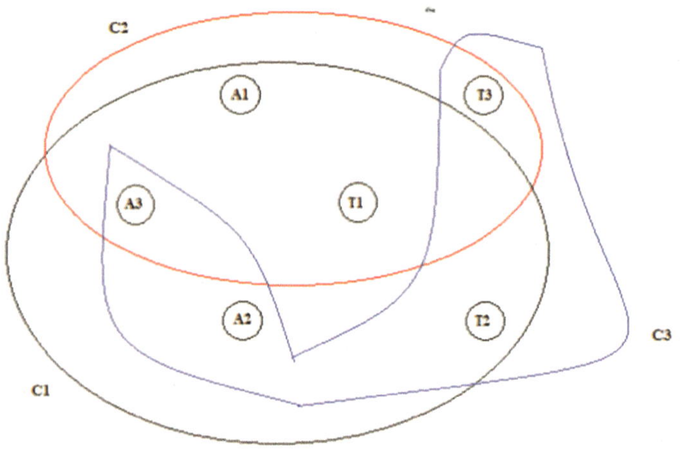

Fig. 15.5 Clusters formed by the vertices in the network

tolerated by the people, it can often obstruct the locals' activities (which are illegal and wrong). The examination of these interactions reveals an essential aspect of the elements' connection. These connections are used to learn more about other areas of technology applications for the protection of wild species [21]. To visualize the relationships between the elements, a graph is built with all of the interacting elements as vertices and the relationships between them as edges [20].

Although the graph in the result part of this study looks to be simple, it would be considerably more thick and intricate in the actual world. This graph also aids in the visualization of inter-set interactions, which may be used to better understand how cooperation among components of the same set can result in differences in net interactions [1]. To investigate the implications, a clique was provided, which demonstrates and validates that all parts of the considered sets interact with one another to form the complex system of tradition vs. technology in the PA's peripheral areas.

Furthermore, the centrality analysis of the network yields a set of clusters based on the weight of the graph's edges, as determined by the game theoretic interaction of the variables [26]. C1, C2 and C3 are the three main clusters that develop. The study of these clusters identifies A_3 as the common factor for all three clusters, which is one of the three aspects of technology deployment. The factor A_3 is linked to the use of fence measures to keep wild animals from entering residential or human areas, as mentioned in the preceding sections. The fences surrounding the agricultural or village boundaries are erected to reduce human-animal conflict and prevent residents from suffering losses because of PA wild animal attacks [24].

The preceding debate reveals an intriguing truth regarding the local inhabitants' perceptions and psychology about technology deployments for the protection of and against wild animals. Although the human footprints in the region may not be conducive to technological deployment for a variety of reasons, when it comes to survival, people must overcome the elements.

The second essential point to note about the proposed model is that, while the interactions and payoffs have been calculated for the ideal situation of maximal cooperation or defection, the model is also area particular. By "area particular," it means the area around the settlements. Nearer to the villages, there is more defection to technology components, which gradually diminishes as we travel further away. The scenario is illustrated in Fig. 15.6 for the model elements A_1, A_2 and A_3 in relation to the hypothetical terrain.

Conclusion

The suggested model in this chapter provides a fundamental computational framework for understanding the relationship between local inhabitants' cognition and the technical instruments used for animal conservation in these protected regions. The study is divided into three sections: (a) game theoretic modelling of interactions, (b) interaction graph building and (c) clustering of the criticals of the interactions.

The author has limited the number of interaction settings in order to keep the work intelligible and self-contained. It has been stated and proposed that while the work may have a variety of parameters, they would all serve as new variables in the model. The ability to arrange technology rollout without harming locals is a vital component of the modelling job. Various approaches have been created in the past for this aim, but they have only partially succeeded in achieving the objectives [29]. The work's originality consists in how villagers' cognition can be comprehended and modelled using various technology aspects so that the best conservation methods may be implemented while taking into consideration local support. Conservation of wild species while retaining local support can be a tough challenge to do simultaneously, but the model described in this chapter takes into consideration maintaining a balance between the two in order to achieve long-term conservation goals. Because they are the first victims of human-animal conflicts, it is critical to obtain local support.

Using the locals' survival behaviour in deploying technology aspects that can be supported and, in many cases, maintained by the locals is one of the most important takeaways from the concept. Understanding how and when to accomplish this is a critical task, and the architecture of the approaches used in this study suggests how the process may be structured and completed effectively.

The model has been kept basic to make it self-sustaining, and all of the experiments are based on ideal interaction conditions. The work's creator claims that in the future, enhancements to the work can be made by integrating more elements. These aspects include a complete survey of the locals, a full field research for the work, parameter mapping utilizing remote sensing and geographic information system techniques, and so on. However, despite its simplicity, the suggested model may always be utilized for technology deployment tasks by expanding the number of variables and including partial interaction scores that are spatial and time dependent.

Fig. 15.6 The interplay of all three-technology deployment factors as a function of distance from residential and human-occupied areas

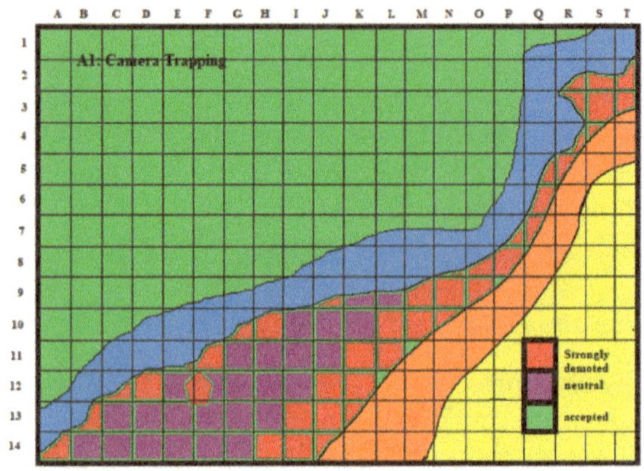

(a) A1: Camera Trapping

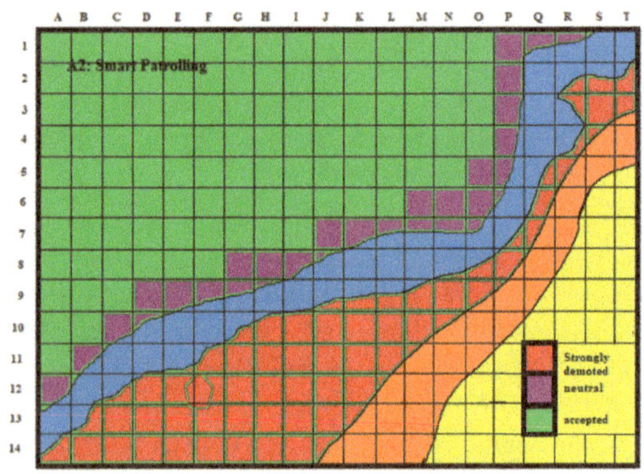

(b) A2: Smart Patrolling

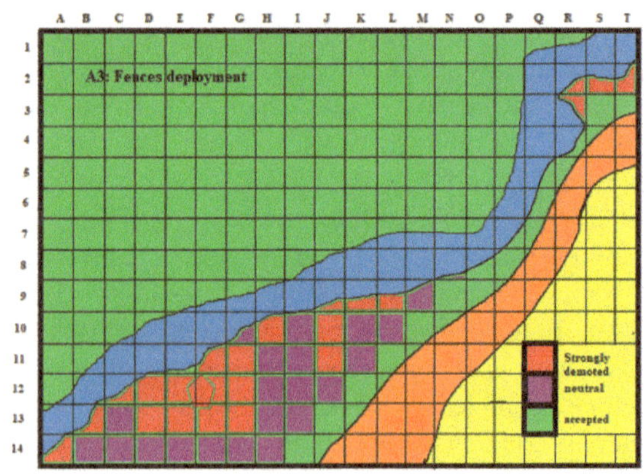

(c) Fences deployment

References

1. Agapito, G., Guzzi, P., Cannataro, M.: Visualization of protein interaction networks: problems and solutions. BMC Bioinf. **14**(Suppl 1), S1 (2013)
2. Albaba, B.M., Yildiz, Y.: Modeling cyber-physical human systems via an interplay between reinforcement learning and game theory. Annu. Rev. Control **48**, 1–21 (2019)
3. Balister, P., Győri, E., Schelp, R.: Coloring vertices and edges of a graph by nonempty subsets of a set. Eur. J. Comb. **32**(4), 533–537 (2011)
4. Cameron, R.P.: Protected area—working forest interface: ecological concerns for protected areas management in Canada. Nat. Areas J. **26**(4), 403–407 (2006)
5. Chakraborty, N., Lukovnikov, D., Maheshwari, G., Trivedi, P., Lehmann, J., Fischer, A.: Introduction to neural network-based question answering over knowledge graphs. WIREs Data Mining Knowl Discovery **11**(3) (2021)
6. Conlon, D.: Graphs with few paths of prescribed length between any two vertices. Bull. Lond. Math. Soc. **51**(6), 1015–1021 (2019)
7. Davis, R.K.: Wildlife and people: the human dimensions of wildlife ecology. In: Gary, G.G. (ed.). Urbana and Chicago: University of Illinois Press, 1993. xii + 260 pp. Illustrations, notes, references, index. $39.95. Forest Conserv. History **38**(4), 198 (1994)
8. Dickman, A.J.: Complexities of conflict: the importance of considering social factors for effectively resolving human-wildlife conflict. Anim. Conserv. **13**(5), 458–466 (2010)
9. Game Theory and Applications: Int. Game Theory Rev. **08**(02), 327 (2006)
10. Hernandez, G., Leon, R., Salinas, L., Dimnet, E.: A fragmentation model with neighborhood interaction. Appl. Math. Model. **36**(4), 1694–1702 (2012)
11. Joseph, K.B., Alexey, V., William, O.: Analysis of human activities in and around protected areas (PAs): case of Kakum conservation area in Ghana. Int. J. Biodivers. Conserv. **6**(7), 541–554 (2014)
12. Kabalak, A., Smirnova, E., Jost, J.: Non-cooperative game theory in biology and cooperative reasoning in humans. Theory Biosci. **134**(1–2), 17–46 (2015)
13. Karlapudy, D.A.M.: IOT based agricultural fields protection from animals. Int. J. Res. Appl. Sci. Eng. Technol. **7**(5), 3086–3090 (2019)
14. Maclean, K.: Seeing, being seen, and not being seen: pilgrimage, tourism, and layers of looking at the kumbh mela. CrossCurrents **59**(3), 319–341 (2009)
15. MacNulty, D.R., Plumb, G.E., Smith, D.W.: Validation of a new video and telemetry system for remotely monitoring wildlife. J. Wildl. Manag. **72**(8), 1834–1844 (2008)
16. Massei, G., Coats, J., Lambert, M.S., Pietravalle, S., Gill, R., Cowan, D.: Camera traps and activity signs to estimate wild boar density and derive abundance indices. Pest Manag. Sci. **74**(4), 853–860 (2017)
17. Meghanathan, N.: A comprehensive analysis of the correlation between maximal clique size and centrality metrics for complex network graphs. Egypt. Inf. J. Published (2016)
18. Nandy, A., Sen, S., Sopena, R.: Outerplanar and planar oriented cliques. J. Graph Theory **82**(2), 165–193 (2015)
19. Protection of Endangered Species of Wild Fauna and Flora (2021). Advances in Earth and Environmental Science. Published
20. SAARINEN, J.: Visual search for positional relationships between pattern elements. Scand. J. Psychol. **37**(3), 294–301 (1996)
21. Seymour, V.: The human–nature relationship and its impact on health: a critical review. Frontiers Public Health **4** (2016)
22. Shanu, S., Idiculla, J., Qureshi, Q., Jhala, Y., Aggarwal, A., Dimri, P., Bhattacharya, S.: A graph theoretic approach for modelling tiger corridor network in Central India-Eastern Ghats landscape complex, India. Eco. Inform. **50**, 76–85 (2019)
23. Sima, V., Gheorghe, I. G., Subić, J., Nancu, D.: Influences of the Industry 4.0 revolution on the human capital development and consumer behavior: a systematic review. Sustainability **12**(10), 4035 (2020)

24. Songhurst, A.: Measuring human-wildlife conflicts: comparing insights from different monitoring approaches. Wildl. Soc. Bull. **41**(2), 351–361 (2017)
25. Sugeng, K.A., Ryan, J.: Clique vertex magic cover of a graph. Math. Comput. Sci. **5**(1), 113–118 (2011)
26. Szczepański, P.L., Michalak, T.P., Rahwan, T.: Efficient algorithms for game-theoretic betweenness centrality. Artif. Intell. **231**, 39–63 (2016)
27. Thompson, P.B.: Designing animals: ethical issues for genetic engineers. J. Dairy Sci. **75**(8), 2294–2303 (1992)
28. Toyoizumi, H.: Evolution of Cooperation on Playing Prisoner's Dilemma Game in the Finite-Capacity Spot. Published, Nature Precedings (2009)
29. Urbanik, A.: Ethnic policy as a subject of social science research. Different theoretical approaches. Wrocławskie Studia Politologiczne **29**, 79–89 (2021)
30. Voss, K.E.: One field, many disciplines, one goal. Am. J. Bioeth. **2**(4), 1–2 (2002). https://doi.org/10.1162/152651602320957411
31. Wix, N., Reich, M.: Time-triggered camera traps versus line transects –advantages and limitations of multi-method studies for bird surveys. Bird Study **66**(2), 207–223 (2019)

Chapter 16
Impact of Disruptive Technologies on Society to Combat Pandemics

Tapalina Bhattasali and Xavier Savarimuthu

Introduction

Disruptive technologies play a significant role to maintain a sustainable society, especially during any disasters like pandemic outbreak. Human race was threatened before by the disasters like SARS, H1N1, and Ebola. These unexpected diseases took away millions of lives. For each such outbreak, people need to learn new ways of fighting. Generally, digital technology can help to prevent the spread of viruses as well as to minimize its impact. In the year 2020, COVID-19 is declared as a global pandemic as corona virus has caused socio-economic crises all over the world. All the countries are affected by COVID-19 pandemic, which adversely affects the existing infrastructure of the society [1, 2]. Advanced digital technologies show a ray of hope in pandemic management. These technologies can provide multi-dimensional benefits.

COVID vaccine delivery including its distribution and management gives rise to several challenges like manufacturing delay, risks of delays in vaccine shipments, prioritization of populations to receive vaccinations, complexity of scheduling vaccinations, tracking recipients. Disruptive technologies enable efficient use of vaccine and healthcare equipment, checkup, and surveillance with minimum human intervention. It is possible to detect the gathering of people from the collected data. Sensors can visualize the production line; smart manufacturing processes can manufacture essential disposable items for pandemic management; and smart supply chains can provide essential items needed to fight against COVID-19. Therefore, it is very much

T. Bhattasali (✉) · X. Savarimuthu
St. Xavier's College (Autonomous), Kolkata, India
e-mail: tapalina@sxccal.edu

X. Savarimuthu
e-mail: envsxavi@sxccal.edu

A. Choudhury et al. (eds.), *Evolution of Digitized Societies Through Advanced Technologies*, Advanced Technologies and Societal Change,
https://doi.org/10.1007/978-981-19-2984-7_16

required to confirm the utility of disruptive technologies for COVID-19 pandemic management.

Advanced technology can be used not only to manage global pandemic but also to restore the global economy. COVID-19 is considered here as a case study. Its impact on society is so rapid that initially people hardly have any time to take necessary actions. At present, emerging technologies provide tools to respond effectively to coronavirus outbreak compared to the previous outbreaks of disease like SARS, MERS, and Ebola. Nowadays, 4G/5G, high speed internet, mobile, cloud, analytics, artificial intelligence, and machine learning like converging technologies are considered to design innovative solutions to combat pandemic outbreak. Although all countries have their own unique way to respond to this crisis, they need to mainly focus on how to sustain the environment in post-COVID era. Initiatives are taken by the governments to tackle various challenges faced due to the rapid spread of corona virus. The outcome of crisis response strategy entirely depends on how policymakers select and use the appropriate technology and its relevant policies to slow-down or stop the rapid spread of corona virus. The immediate requirement is to break the transmission chain as early as possible. Although healthcare professionals [3–5], government officials, and social workers are the main front-line warriors, the role of information and communication technology is to support them in their work, to provide them new ways to proceed further quickly and accurately. In the present scenario, people who are working at the front-line to save the communities from COVID-19 pandemic, frequently become the carrier of the virus. Humans should not step out in containment zones because of the quick spread of virus from human to human. Therefore, it is very challenging to reach to the public, to supply essential goods to the self-isolated people, or to deliver medical treatment to high-risk areas like hospitals. As a solution, humans need to delegate the responsibilities to machines to sustain in this pandemic. The motto of the society in this crisis period should be to "stay alert-stay safe-stay connected with the digital services". Start of vaccination drives around the world now raises hopes for a global recovery of pandemics. The objective of this chapter is to focus on how the world can use disruptive technologies to respond to the pandemic and the crisis due to it.

Technology to Fight Again COVID-19

Digital Technology is playing a crucial role in keeping society sustainable during COVID-19 pandemic. This pandemic crisis has accelerated the need for automation in every industry to avoid human interaction. Autonomous vehicles like driverless cars, drones, and robots can help in everyday life during this global pandemic by delivering foods and medicines, transporting people while maintaining social distance. Disruptive technologies have the capability to provide better digital solutions for day-to-day crises. Digitized solutions can be considered to provide sustainable solutions without imposing any risk to healthcare workers [6–9]. Robotic based solutions can be considered for infected patients to reduce risk. During the lockdown, people can do their daily work with the help of digital technologies. Medical equipment and precautionary items are manufactured and supplied in time using smart technologies in the supply chain.

Advanced digital technologies make it possible to provide telemedicine service for remote areas. Abnormality of the patients can be detected and informed immediately to medical practitioners. Digital technologies are helpful for virtual classrooms during COVID-19 pandemic. During the lockdown, teaching–learning also becomes possible in remote areas. Disruptive technologies are also termed as Industry 4.0 technologies, which can identify COVID-19 symptoms, and relevant health issues. These technologies are also used to predict expected chances of recovery. AI-based video surveillance can help to observe COVID affected patients and reduce workload of medical practitioners. Artificial intelligence is used to identify fake news on COVID-19 spread through various online platforms.

Emerging technologies like artificial intelligence (AI) are being deployed to monitor and implement solutions to combat the pandemic. As the demand for digital services is increasing day by day, several technological solutions have been developed for allocating resources, tracking infection, screening population, managing communication, and responses. AI is an efficient tool to deal with the outbreak situation of global pandemics. AI techniques can be used to understand the spreading pattern of viruses. Collected data is analyzed using algorithms on artificial intelligence, machine-learning, and natural language processing to predict its impact in global scenarios. Government can take necessary steps to sustain in the event of an emergency. An analysis of the COVID-19 outbreak will prepare the environment for such situations in future. AI is also playing a vital role in finding COVID-19 vaccine. Here technology is used to understand protein structures of the virus for suggesting components of the vaccine. AI-based risk assessment tools can be used to clarify the confusion caused by corona virus. As AI tools can differentiate between common cold or flu and COVID-19 case, it can easily be decided whether the individual needs to be tested or which type of test is suitable for the individual [10–12].

To avoid human contract, autonomous vehicles like self-driving cars can transport COVID positive patients to and fro hospital without affecting other people. Robots, self-driving cars, and trucks can deliver daily needs like meals, groceries, and medical supplies. Removing the human driver reduces the risks of riders to be affected by viruses in these uncertain times [13, 14].

In automated contact tracing, behavioral analytics is used to create social interaction graphs by evaluating data collected from citizens such as location of mobile phones, interaction details, facial recognition, gatherings they attended, and other relevant information. Figure 16.1 represents the basic concept of contact tracing.

Table 16.1 represents the significance of a few major disruptive technologies.

There are a number of bots that can screen people to record vital information, check symptoms, assist people with COVID-19 symptoms on behalf of doctors, and pass the information to doctors only if the condition is critical. To reduce the administrative burden on a limited number of healthcare personnel and staff, AI-based chat-bots and robot-advisory services are used. Bots can also be deployed in rural areas or largest slum areas for mass testing to prevent the spread. Use of robots

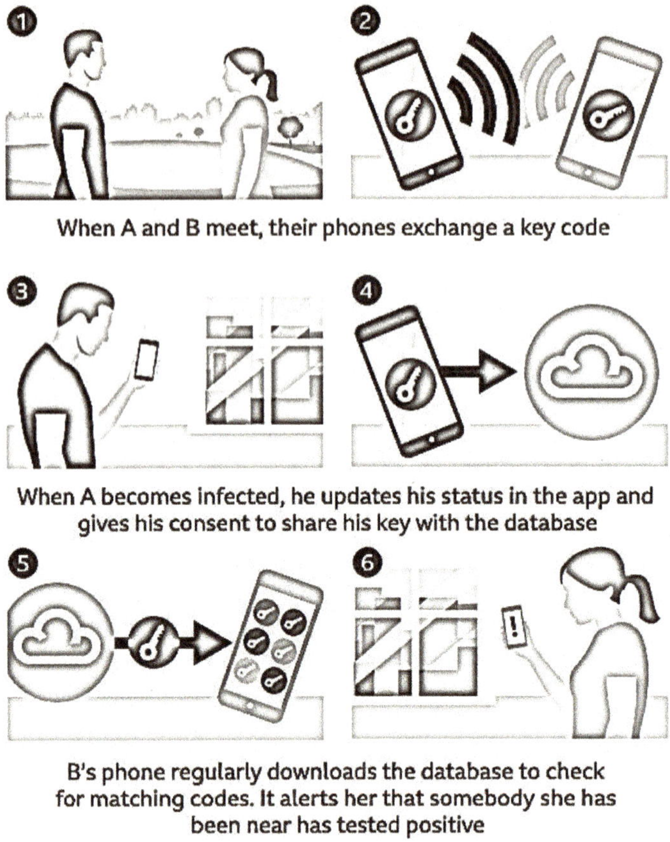
1
2
When A and B meet, their phones exchange a key code
3
4
When A becomes infected, he updates his status in the app and gives his consent to share his key with the database
5
6
B's phone regularly downloads the database to check for matching codes. It alerts her that somebody she has been near has tested positive

Fig. 16.1 Concept of contact tracing

can reduce the probability of human exposure. Robots are being used for jobs such as sanitizing hospitals, measuring body temperature, delivering food, grocery, cooking means and medicines to the patients, and patrolling the streets all over the world. In the present "touch-me-not" environment, the drone management system is one of the efficient tools to mitigate COVID-19. As remotely piloted devices, drones are naturally effective to minimize human interactions. Many cities are using drones for delivering food, carrying medical kits to quarantine areas, monitoring people to enforce social distancing, tracking populations, spraying disinfectant, and using thermal imaging to identify infected people. Police forces have deployed drones for surveillance of public spaces. Drones provide real-time intelligence, which is very much useful as it reduces response time. Command and Control Centre gets immediate notification to send ground force to the incident site for taking necessary actions, in case of any anomalies observed. Drones are also beneficial in preventing theft and unlawful activities.

Table 16.1 Significance of disruptive technologies

Technology	Significance
Artificial Intelligence (AI)	AI can predict outbreak to minimize spread of virus. Fake news in social networks related to COVID-19 can be detected and removed. Optimization of clinical trials for drugs and vaccines can be possible. AI-based robots can automate jobs like helping in sanitization, conducting online medical examinations. It can detect pneumonia through CT scans. It is beneficial to manufacture medical equipment
Robotics	During lockdown, robots are deployed to check whether people are following lockdown orders or not. Hospitals can use robotics to reduce workloads and risks of medical staff without any disruption and to improve the performance
Big Data	It can analyze and forecast the impact of the pandemics on society. Better decisions can be taken by COVID-19 trackers to combat pandemics from the data collected in real-time
Internet of Things (IoT)	Drones can be used to ensure protocols of mask-wearing and quarantine rules are followed by the public. It can trace the origin of the outbreak. It can be used to identify persons who have met infected patients. It can ensure compliance of quarantine by the people. Persons who breach quarantine rules can be identified. It can reduce the load of medical staff by providing facilities of remote health monitoring
Cloud Computing	During social isolation, people can be connected digitally with each other and continue their work with the help of cloud-based applications like Zoom, Google Cloud, Netflix
Biosensors	Biosensors used in glucose monitors can do clinical analysis and diagnose disease accurately. It is very useful for early detection and monitoring of COVID-19 symptoms. Biosensors can record real data of respiration rate, temperature, ECG etc.
Virtual Reality (VR)	It offers facilities for video calls. It makes people feel that they are together without traveling outside. It is an excellent tool for communication and collaboration. VR improves efficiency of working in a group, lowers impact of the environment, reduces travel costs and absenteeism
Holography	It provides facilities to conduct online events. It reduces the possibility of human exposure. It seems that resource persons are virtually alive, which provides ultra-realism. Holography provides the best option for steaming real events during work from home
3D-Printing	3D-Printing can be used to produce face masks that can be used to detect COVID positive quickly. 3D-printed masks can be reused as it is recyclable
3D-Scanning	It is a non-contact technique, which is used for chest scanning. Virtual reality is the application of this technology

Heat map technology can be used to track hot spots and anticipates locations with increasing coronavirus infection rates. Data algorithms and predictive analytics identify geographical areas that are likely to be affected. Heat map is created where dark blue or dark red areas are used to visualize the highest concentration of infections. This feature can be used to improve PPE supply chain management and keep staff safe. As it can predict the next hotspot areas of infection, it is easier to decide how PPE can be mobilized to those geographic areas faster compared to other areas. The heat map is developed from a number of responses collected from Facebook surveys, and the spread of the virus can be monitored by Google users.

Sensor technology is being used in designing disposable, protective face masks that would generate signals if the wearer is infected with the novel Corona virus. Fluorescent signal is produced by this type of facemask when a COVID positive person breathes, coughs, or sneezes.

Big data analytics can be used in pandemic management by quickly identifying infected individuals, monitoring them to track people who came in contact with them.

Facial recognition technologies can verify the identity of people accurately even if they are wearing face-masks. Quarantined people can be easily tracked by monitoring their movement. It also keeps track of people to verify whether they are in contact with an infected person or not. CCTV cameras can identify infected people who break the quarantine rules and go outside during the isolation period along with facial recognition technologies. Table 16.2 represents the merits and demerits of a few major features required for fighting against this pandemic along with technology behind it.

Infrared body temperature measuring devices along with wireless thermometer guns are being used at checkpoints of various public places like hospitals, airports, offices, shops, hotels, and train stations. Individuals who need further investigation can easily be identified while measuring body-temperature from a distance [15–17]. The overall procedure becomes faster and more effective if facial recognition is used along with an automated thermal monitoring system. Misinformation or fake news related to COVID-19 can only create panic and anxiety among the mass-population which in turn results in unwanted scenarios. To reduce false information, companies like Google and Facebook are guiding people with right information provided by WHO, government, or local authorities. Citizens can join an authorized WhatsApp group to clear their doubts. The aim here is to create a transparent scenario where confusion among the citizens is reduced. Trending technologies are used to provide visibility of the outbreak, clear message, status report, and appropriate precautions to the citizens.

Remote working technologies are used to support social distancing as well as to maintain business continuity and economic growth. Features like cloud conferencing, virtual meeting, online platform for education, virtual or augmented reality, secure access to data, enterprise application become very popular to continue regular work-schedule from home during lockdown.

Digital technologies play a significant role in planning, delivery, monitoring, and management of COVID vaccination drives. There are many tools being considered to support vaccination. Many countries use open source platforms for new

Table 16.2 Merits and Demerits of Major Features

Features	Digital technology	Merits	Demerits
Contact tracing	Global positioning systems; mobile phone applications; real-time monitoring of mobile devices; wearable technology	Identifies exposed individuals for testing and quarantine; tracks viral spread	Privacy can be breached; individuals who have not been exposed but have had contact can also be detected; if application is deactivated or mobile device is unavailable or Wi-Fi or cell connectivity is inadequate, individuals who are exposed cannot be detected
Tracking	Machine learning; data dashboards; real-time data from smartphones and wearable technology	Allows visual depiction of spread; guides resource allocation; informs forecasts	Could breach privacy; involves high costs;
Quarantine	Artificial intelligence; cameras and digital recorders; mobile phone applications; global positioning systems (GPS); quick response codes	Isolates infections; restricts travel	Civil liberties are violated; access to food and essential services may be restricted; individuals violating quarantine rules cannot be detected without devices
Clinical management	Artificial intelligence for diagnostics; machine learning; virtual care or telemedicine platforms	Assists with clinical decision-making, diagnostics, and risk prediction; facilitates patient-centered, remote care; facilitates infection control	Could breach privacy; fails to accurately diagnose patients; involves high costs; equipment may malfunction

registration and decision support systems. Existing digital tools can be deployed to track movement of stocks of COVID-19 vaccines. Digital recording of vaccination and follow-up systems using reliable unique identification of the population can determine eligibility and track patients between doses.

Global Scenarios

Different parts of the world are using different technologies to prevent loss of life, to minimize the negative impact of enormous socio-economic disruption amidst pandemic outbreak.

South Korea uses the concept of robotics to maintain social distancing amidst of corona virus. A self-driven robot along with LED screen and cameras can welcome people in the office lobby, check their temperature, and dispense hand sanitizer. Data can be transmitted to its server in real-time using 5G technology. Robot raises alarm if temperature is more than 99.5-degree Fahrenheit. It can warn people in the group to maintain physical distance. It reminds people to wear facemask. To protect privacy of the visitors it can hide face of the visitors mirrored in the screen. Artificial Intelligence is used here to increase accuracy of temperature measurement and to reduce time. Robot can disinfect 99% surface area quickly using ultraviolet lamps and disinfectant sprayers. In the cafe, robots are used as waiters to take food orders. These robots can prepare different types of drinks and serve at the seats of the customers. In multiplex cinema hall, robots can be used to sell movie tickets, parking vouchers, and popcorns. They can also guide customers to their seats at cinema hall or toilet. Self-driving food-delivery robot Delitower can either pick up food from the restaurants or delivery riders to deliver foods at the location of customer, who places food-order through QR code.

In Hong Kong, use of electronic wristbands is mandatory to enforce self-isolation. In the StayHomeSafe app, the user needs to scan the unique QR code to pair the wristband with the smartphone app. This technique is used to ensure that people who have recent travel history stay at home. It can reduce the probability of spreading the virus. For densely populated cities like Hong Kong, where GPS cannot work effectively, Geo-fencing technique is used to create a virtual perimeter for real-world geographic areas. As the quarantined resident walks around the apartment, the app creates composite signature to track the coordinates of the living space by sampling the signals and wristband is calibrated accordingly. The app triggers a warning to the Government for taking necessary steps, if any person leaves the quarantine place. Quarantined people can use delivery apps for ordering food and groceries.

Taiwan has also deployed tracking technology to enforce quarantine measures. During this global pandemic, cellular signals on phones are considered to monitor the location and movements of people. Taiwan builds a monitoring system to provide real-time alerts by combining health data with the travel data. For example, automated alerts are sent if people have travelled to the infected vicinity.

Advanced digital infrastructure and engineering capabilities of Singapore enables the government to tackle COVID-19 outbreak quickly in an efficient manner. The necessary information required to manage the crisis is transmitted quickly and accurately to the citizens by using a suite of digital tools. The Singapore government identifies COVID-19 positive patients and isolates them immediately and uses contract tracing to identify suspected persons. Suspected persons are served with "Stay Home Notice (SHN)" for fourteen days. Smart-phones along with video and voice calls,

GPS tracking can monitor people regularly during self-isolation periods. If isolated persons violate quarantine orders, they will be punished. SHN users need to submit videos or photos of their surroundings. Text messages are sent to the users with a link containing a GPS location request, which needs to be clicked within 60 min, so that authorities can visit the place without any notifications. Activities of SHN users can also be analyzed from their mobile phone logs and surveillance video cameras. Bluetooth application can also be used to enable more efficient contact tracing, which is very significant to incorporate safe distancing rules in public places and for enforcing compulsory quarantine for incoming travellers.

Contact tracing mobile app TraceTogether is used to mitigate the spread of COVID-19 through Bluetooth signals. Installed app in one mobile can detect proximity of other phones. Consequently, distance between users and duration of contact can be determined. Digital records are locally stored in encrypted format on each user's phone. Authorized users can upload TraceTogether data to the Ministry of Health (MoH), which are decrypted to retrieve the contact numbers of the close contacts. This enables identification of close contacts of confirmed cases more quickly.

AI-driven automated temperature screening gantry VigilantGantry can enhance rate of contactless screening along with saving manpower and time. Abnormal temperature is quickly detected, and alert is generated. This is very useful for detection of symptomatic cases. Modular VigilantGantry can be easily integrated with existing thermal systems, mobile optical cameras, and facial recognition solutions for contact tracing.

GovTech developed an automated temperature scanner to do a temperature scan before entering into a building or office. This system can be considered in any Government Buildings and community facilities. GovTech also developed cloud-based visitor registration system, where visitors scan QR code using SingPass mobile app and give consent to share their name and contact information along with necessary declaration. This service is regularly updated to provide the latest guidelines.

Virtual assistant AskJamie is designed to answer queries. Chatbots are used to address queries related to COVID-19, and machine learning algorithms are used to improve accuracy of the replies. Trending topics are identified by data analytics tools. Citizens can also access chatbots via Facebook Messenger and Telegram. Biz chatbot addresses business related questions in the context of COVID-19.

SMS and web-based solution Leave of Absence and Stay-Home Notice Tracking Solution allows people to report their locations to the Ministry of Manpower quickly and accurately. The FluGoWhere website provides special subsidies for patients having respiratory problems. Official WhatsApp account gov.sg provides trusted updates on the COVID-19 pandemic in a timely manner. These updates are available in different languages. Citizens need to register to subscribe to the updates.

MaskGoWhere website helps Singaporean households to find the allotted schedule and their allotted mask collection location. GovTech has made progressive updates and improvements to the website based on the latest available information and insights gathered through real-time user feedback. The Singapore government set up a dedicated WhatsApp channel for interacting with all the residents in the context of their mental and physical well-being.

During the pandemic, China Government has made it mandatory to provide personal data to access public services. Topmost telecom companies send bulk text messages to provide customer information about the cities they have visited in the past 15 or 30 days. The information is being used to restrict movement. Railway stations and residential neighborhoods use this type of information to allow required passengers and residents to enter.

In the cities like Shanghai and Shenzhen, citizens need to declare their identities on a phone app to avail city subway service like riding in a train. This app can easily monitor the close contacts of the users to track whether users come close to the affected or suspected persons or not. Identity verification procedures can also work in cinema halls, where movie-goers need to provide their personal details to book their seats.

In Baidu, an AI-based solution is used for screening large populations effectively. This system can examine about 200 people per minute without any disruption in normal work and detect changes in body temperature of people while they are moving. It can be incorporated in crowded areas, airports, rail stations, hospitals to identify COVID positive people quickly, and quarantine them before they infect a larger population.

Social media platforms like TikTok in association with WHO provide their users with correct, timely facts on COVID-19, along with a live stream from the WHO, where users can ask questions and seek answers.

Messaging service WeChat uses color based QR codes determine how safe a person is. Based on personal and location data three-color code is generated. Green indicates person is safe, yellow indicates person needs seven-day quarantine, and red indicates fourteen-day quarantine. This feature enables authorities to track movements of people over time as the user's location along with identifying code number has been sent to the server connected to the police.

CRUZR robot is a user-friendly companion in the hospital to reduce the workload of major staff in hospital. It can perform basic tasks such as body temperature checking. The WHISPIR platform in Australia allows business and Government agencies to send messages to citizens regarding a variety of actions required to keep track of the quarantined people. Isolated persons need to respond to a series of questions to confirm their conditions.

In Australia, Telestra Health helps to deliver connectivity required for tele-health appointments. Remote monitoring gear collects blood pressure, pulse, and oxygen saturation readings with SpO_2 pulse oximeters from low-risk COVID-19 patients in their homes. Collections are forwarded to large public hospitals or emergency departments. Its objective is to provide adequate medical care and support to self-isolators as well as to reduce the probability of infectious patients to go outside. At the same time, the Australian Government has initiated fast tracking of implementation of electronic prescriptions. It results in faster delivery medicare benefit policy compared to pre-COVID environment.

Message Manager software reports healthcare progress to residents and their families by using communication and record management facilities. Covidsafe app is used to automate COVID-19 contact tracing.

Africans have designed mobile technology solutions to control the pandemic. In Nigeria, online COVID-19 Triage Tool is used to self-assess the risk category of corona virus. Interactive chat service about coronavirus has been provided by the government through WhatsApp. In Africa, mobile technology solutions are used in various ways from WhatsApp Chabot to self-diagnosis tools to combat COVID-19.

Indian Scenarios

Different states in India are focusing on different solutions to tackle COVID-19 such as thermal cameras for fever detection, drones-based surveillance for crowd monitoring, and Chabot for emergency e-pass system. Smart cities in India are using GIS to map each COVID-19 positive case, GPS to track health care workers, and heat mapping technologies to draw containment plans. Smart technology solutions are used to help administration to manage complex civic functions and law and order of the society. There is a seamless integration among technologies in monitoring and managing crowds, delivering messages, tracking patients, and communicating with the citizens. Police agencies use technology to manage command and control centers or city operation centers. Peer to peer communication is going on via intercom, mobile phone, and videoconferencing. In India, telecom companies like BSNL, airtel, and Jio are spreading awareness of pandemic through the caller tunes. There are a number of mobile apps launched by the Government of India to make lives of citizens easier amidst of COVID-19. There is a contact-tracing mobile app Arogya Setu designed in eleven languages to help citizens to identify their risk of contracting the novel coronavirus. It uses location data of smart phones and Bluetooth to verify whether users meet a COVID infected person or not. This app shares data of the users to the Government if they come close to COVID positive persons.

BHIM UPI app can be used to initiate cashless payment for touchless transactions for a range of utility services required during the isolation period. Umang app provides more than 600 major utility services provided by central and state government departments or other private organizations such as Aadhar, passport, driving license, PAN, and PF. Ayush Sanjivani app aims to create awareness regarding Ayush advocacies and measures its usage among the population and its impact in the prevention of Corona virus. Jan Aushadi Sugam app provides details about the availability and pricing of generic medicines sold at lower prices. It can also locate the nearest center from where medicines can be purchased. E-Gram Swaraj app is used for rural development across the nation. Government can easily reach rural people to identify their needs through this e-governance model.

In India, the robots are initially used to reduce the chance of hospital staff to be affected by the virus [18–21]. At the early stage of this global pandemic, Kerala emerged as a role model in India for fighting against COVID-19. In Kerala, Asimov

Robotics deployed robots that can distribute masks, tissue papers, and sanitizers; disinfect door handles and play videos that can help to create awareness on COVID-19 pandemic. Robots can also answer queries on COVID-19. In Ernakulum, an inexpensive robot Karmi-Bot has been designed that can disinfect hospitals using UV rays and carry food and medical supplies to the patients in isolation wards. In Tamil Nadu, a 4 ft. tall Zafi robot can carry payload up to 8 kgs with a Wi-Fi connection range of 250 m. This robot can reach patients in isolation wards and patients can collect food when the robot rings the bell after reaching outside the rooms. Patients can talk with healthcare personnel or clear their doubts through communication and voice-interaction mechanisms fitted within the robot. Zafi-med robot can be operated from a distance of 1.5 km, and it can carry loads up to 20 kgs to deliver essentials to the home-quarantined people. In Bengaluru, Invento Robotics has designed an autonomous robot Astra that can disinfect quarantine rooms and hospitals using powerful UVC (ultraviolet light spectrum) to kill most of the bacteria and viruses including Corona virus. Table 16.3 represents major technology solutions in different states.

Government of India scales up drone monitoring to enforce ban on religious or any other type of gathering. All states in India are mandatorily disinfecting contaminated areas to prevent the spread of virus. However, it is difficult for the Government to manage it in the traditional way due to rapid transmission of viruses. Unmanned vehicles become key tools in the Corona virus battle. The drones like Marut can be used for spraying disinfectants in public areas like parks, airports, railway stations, etc. Drones can disinfect 50 times more area within a given time than traditional methods. It also reduces human intervention to keep them safe. Police in many states like Telengana, Delhi, West Bengal, and Maharashtra have used drones to ensure full lockdown is maintained in the town. Fly base drones can deliver emergency supplies, medicines, first-aid kits to homes and hospitals, send live video to COVID-19 centers,

Table 16.3 Major technology solutions at different states

States	Technology to combat COVID-19
Maharashtra	Crowd Monitoring, Smart Operators, Public Messaging, Mobile Command Centre, Vehicle Monitoring
Rajasthan	Crowd and Vehicle Monitoring, COVID-19 helpline
Gujrat	Crowd Control
Uttar Pradesh	City Operations Centre, COVID-19 helpline, Variable Message Display, Smart Meter
Chattisgarh	COVID Command Centre, Variable Message Display
Odisha	Curfew Warning: Early Warning Dissemination System
Telengana	AI-based Vehicle Movement Monitoring, AI-based Crowd Control, Public Messaging & Variable Message Display, Robots
Tamil Nadu	24*7 Operations of Tamil Nadu State Data Centre, Robots
Andhra-Pradesh	24 * 7 COViD-19 Contact Centre, Public Messaging, COVID-19 Survey, Citizens App with COVID-19 SoS Button

spray disinfectants, monitor the public for crowd control, and warn people regarding the requirements of staying inside home. Drones or night-vision drones fly for a radius of 2–3 km to monitor hotspot locations in the city both in the morning and the evening. Drones can reduce the probability of the danger where front-line fighters like health workers are easily infected. Drones also help us in ensuring that there is ample social distancing between the crowds queuing up in front of pharmacies and grocery stores. Authorities can ensure safety of their personnel while monitoring a larger area and incorporating social distancing in a lesser time.

To ensure that citizens in Hyderabad are not going beyond three kilometers from their residence for any reason as per order, an automated number plate recognition system is designed based on machine-learning algorithms. Crowd analytics triggers real-time alerts to help police to disperse the crowd.

In Bihar, the disaster management department has developed a Garur app to help Government officials and health professionals for monitoring international and national travelers. This app can identify the persons who have recently entered Bihar and analyze their travel history to trace whether they have come from different countries or from different states of India. It not only helps the Government to trace the migrants but also makes it possible to provide shelter and required food.

During the lockdown period, many migrants in India are moving to their hometowns by foot due to lack of transport. Many of them died because of having no shelter or food in their route. Google India has added a new feature to its search engine, assistant, and maps to display lists of night shelters and food shelters in many Corona virus affected Indian cities. Although Google has started this feature in English, it will soon be available in Hindi or other local languages to make it more user-friendly for the migrant workers. Beside this, Google India is trying to build various solutions that help people during their need. Relevant information during this crisis period has been conveyed to the affected people, who cannot afford smartphones. Professors of IIT Roorkee have developed an app as a surveillance system for tracking suspected patients. This app can create geo-fencing around the quarantined person. If geo-fencing is violated, the system or concerned authorities will receive alerts. In any case, if GPS data is not available, the information related to location will be obtained by triangulation of mobile towers. Location will be notified through SMS when Internet is not available. Immediate alert will be generated when the application terminates abruptly. Quarantined persons need to share their photos and places in Google map randomly; so that administrators can view all reports on a map and track the entire movement history of an individual. This app can provide the history of all people in the vicinity of the affected person for a certain period. Besides providing quarantine management service, this app can issue alerts to avoid overcrowding at any place.

Performance of work from home employees can be monitored amid COVID-19 crisis using various software packages. It is to ensure that the work-from-home strategy is not affected during office-hours because of personal issues at home.

Conclusion

COVID-19 pandemic is more devastating and has already killed many people. Policymakers understand that they were not geared up for this pandemic crisis. They need to apply this experience and be prepared in advance against the next pandemic situation to avoid any type of loss for individuals as well as society. Disruptive Technologies are becoming enablers to make the pandemic response faster. These digital technologies play a significant role to combat COVID-19 pandemic. As COVID-19 is a global crisis, advanced digital technologies can provide global standard solutions of the problems. These technologies provide automated solutions. Digital technologies can efficiently isolate infected patients to reduce risk of mortality, improve speed of treatment, and drug manufacturing process. Digitization of society enables people to work from home. They experience a new work culture with a virtual office. These smart technologies provide better crowd management and public safety. Concept of a virtual clinic through telemedicine consultation reduces the possibility of physical crowding of patients.

Digitization has a significant role in society. Lifestyle of people has been transformed from offline to online mode to survive in society. Technologies will continue to advance exponentially. Societies need to adapt to the change and design digital solutions to combat any uncontrolled disasters like pandemics. After COVID-19 outbreak, technological innovation proved its impact on pandemic management and to fight for future emergencies in a timely and systematic manner.

References

1. Javaid, M., Haleem, A.: Industry 4.0 applications in the medical field: a brief review. Curr. Med. Res. Pract. **9**(3), 102e9 (2019)
2. Ienca, M., Vayena, E.: On the responsible use of digital data to tackle the COVID19 pandemic. Nat. Med. **27**, 1e2 (2020)
3. Zeng, J., Huang, J., Pan, L.: How to balance acute myocardial infarction and COVID19: the protocols from Sichuan Provincial People's Hospital. Intensive Care Med. **11**, 1e3 (2020)
4. Manogaran, G., Thota, C., Lopez, D., Sundarasekar, R.: Big Data Security Intelligence for Healthcare Industry 4.0. Cyber Security for Industry, 4.0. Springer, Cham (2017), pp. 103–126
5. Ruan, Q., Yang, K., Wang, W., Jiang, L., Song, J.: Clinical predictors of mortality due to COVID-19 based on an analysis of data of 150 patients from Wuhan, China. Intensive Care Med. **3**, 1e3 (2020)
6. Haleem, A., Javaid, M., Vaishya, R.: Industry 4.0 and its applications in orthopaedics. J. Clin. Orthop. Trauma **10**(3), 615e6 (2019)
7. Cheng, G.J., Liu, L.T., Qiang, X.J., Liu, Y.: Industry 4.0 development and application of intelligent manufacturing. In: 2016 International Conference on Information System and Artificial Intelligence (ISAI). IEEE (2016), pp. 407–410
8. Grasselli, G., Pesenti, A., Cecconi, M.: Critical care utilisation for the COVID-19 outbreak in Lombardy, Italy: early experience and forecast during an emergency response. Jama (2020)
9. Ahmed, S.F., Quadeer, A.A., McKay, M.R.: Preliminary identification of potential vaccine targets for the COVID-19 coronavirus (SARS-CoV-2) based on SARSCoV immunological studies. Viruses **12**(3), 254 (2020 Mar)

10. Haleem, A., Javaid, M.: Additive manufacturing applications in industry 4.0: a review. J. Ind. Integat. Manag. (2019). S2424862219300011
11. Ren, J.L., Zhang, A.H., Wang, X.J.: Traditional Chinese medicine for COVID-19 treatment. Pharmacol. Res. **4**, 104743 (2020 Mar)
12. Alloghani, M., Al-Jumeily, D., Hussain, A., Aljaaf, A.J., Mustafina, J., Petrov, E.: Healthcare services innovations based on the state-of-the-art technology trend industry 4.0. In: 2018 11th International Conference on Developments in eSystems Engineering (DeSE) (2018), pp. 64–70
13. Haleem, A., Javaid, M., Vaishya, R.: Effects of COVID 19 pandemic in daily life. Curr. Med. Res. Pract. (2020). https://doi.org/10.1016/j.cmrp.2020.03.011
14. Fisher, D., Wilder-Smith, A.: The global community needs to swiftly ramp up the response to contain COVID-19. Lancet (London, England) **395**(10230), 1109 (2020 Apr 4)
15. Li, Q., Feng, W., Quan, Y.H.: Trend and forecasting of the COVID-19 outbreak in China. J. Infect. **80**(4), 469–496 (2020 Apr 1)
16. Petropoulos Georgios. Artificial intelligence in the fight against COVID-19. Available from: https://www.bruegel.org/2020/03/artificialintelligence-in-the-fight-against-covid-19/
17. Bean Randy. Big data in the time of coronavirus (COVID-19). Available from: https://www.forbes.com/sites/ciocentral/2020/03/30/big-data-in-the-time-of-coronavirus-covid-19/#161ff87558fc
18. He S. Using the Internet of Things to fight virus outbreaks. Available from: https://www.technologynetworks.com/immunology/articles/usingthe-internet-of-things-to-fight-virus-outbreaks-331992
19. Lawrence C. Is cloud computing the superhero of covid-19? Dev Hub 2020 Mar; Available from: https://www.codemotion.com/magazine/dev-hub/cloud-manager/cloud-computing-covid-19/
20. Baldwin, R., Tomiura, E.: Thinking ahead about the trade impact of COVID-19. Economics in the time of COVID-19 (2020), p. 59
21. Haleem, A., Javaid, M., Vaishya, R., Deshmukh, S.G.: Areas of academic research with the impact of COVID-19. AJEM (Am. J. Emerg. Med.) (2020). https://doi.org/10.1016/j.ajem.2020.04.022